Outpatients
The Astonishing
New World of
Medical Tourism

COLUMBIA GLOBAL REPORTS

NEW YORK

Outpatients
The Astonishing New World of Medical Tourism

Sasha Issenberg

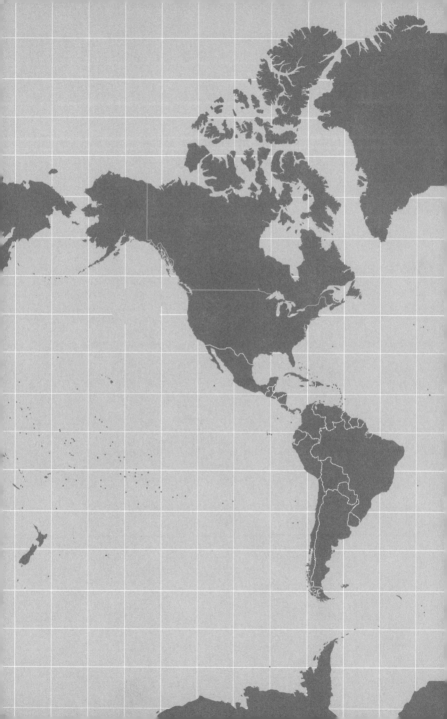

United Kingdom

London

Mosonmagyaróvár

Hungary

Sopron   Budapest

Sofia

Turkey

Japan

Bulgaria

Israel

Thailand

Bangkok

© 2015 Jeffrey L. Ward

Outpatients:
The Astonishing New World of Medical Tourism
Copyright © 2016 by Sasha Issenberg

Published by Columbia Global Reports
91 Claremont Avenue, Suite 515
New York, NY 10027
globalreports.columbia.edu
facebook.com/columbiaglobalreports
@columbiaGR

Library of Congress Control Number: 2015949774
ISBN: 978-0-9909763-8-7

Book design: Strick&Williams
Cover illustrations:
Crown © mustafahacalaki/DigitalVision Vectors/Getty Images
Stamp shapes © edge69/DigitalVision Vectors/Getty Images
Stethoscope © fairywong/DigitalVision Vectors/Getty Images
Heart © Rakdee Phakhasup/DigitalVision Vectors/Getty Images
Baby and Bones © lushik/DigitalVision Vectors/Getty Images
Map design: Jeffrey L. Ward
Author photograph: Akiko Horiyama

Printed in the United States of America

CONTENTS

10
Prologue

19
Chapter One
Orbán's Dentist

27
Chapter Two
Bismarck and Beveridge

37
Chapter Three
Torn Curtain

52
Chapter Four
Brain Drain

68
Chapter Five
Flying Bodies

75
Chapter Six
Europa

86
Chapter Seven
The Bulgarian Method

95
Chapter Eight
The Eastern Front

106
Epilogue

114
Acknowledgments

118
Further Readings

120
Endnotes

To Olga Issenberg, whose love and strength made everything possible for her grandson, including a return to the land of her birth under such curious circumstances

Prologue

The Tokushukai Medical Corporation operates more than 280 hospitals in Japan, enough for the company to often find itself described as the world's largest hospital chain. In 2006, Tokushukai opened its first overseas facility, in Bulgaria, and I had been prepared for its incongruity amid the dreary blocks south of Sofia's downtown. "If you drive there, you will drive through a really bad area, then you see there is some kind of an island," Robert Gerl, the Munich-based CEO of the Bavaria International Health Association, told me. Indeed, the Tokuda Hospital Sofia did stand out from a distance— a nine-story ivory puzzle piece in a sort of corporatized-Bauhaus style—although indoors there was little besides Japanese prints adorning random corridors to distinguish its unusual heritage.

It wasn't until I walked through the orthopedics ward that I fully appreciated what kind of incongruity was possible within the modern hospital. Part of the reason Tokushukai officials had selected the Sofia site was the promise of serving patients throughout the region, but Tokuda began drawing them from other continents as well. Eastern Europe was becoming a destination for Middle Eastern knees, and Tokuda became popular with patients from Oman, one of several Persian Gulf states suffering from abnormally frequent joint injuries. (The culprits appear to be stress from repeated bending at prayer, along with the high rates of non-fatal car accidents that typically accompany a country's belated motorization.)

During a tour of the facility, a hospital staffer mentioned to me the significant number of knee surgery patients from Libya. As Libya's civil war raged on, the country's already limited medical system became even more overcrowded, and Tokuda contracted with authorities there to receive their patients. The staffer gestured toward an open door, and when I poked my head past the threshold, my eyes met those of a woman tucked into the bed, and then those of a man I assumed to be her husband hunched over her. His hand clasped hers, a gesture of comfort that appeared unable to weaken the uncertain fear frozen on her face. A head covering suggested the expectation of modesty, which I was clearly in the midst of defying. I didn't know what to say, or in what language I would possibly say it, and neither did she. I moved along, wordlessly, steadied by the relief that I could not be the source of her anxiety. Here was a Libyan woman trapped in a Japanese hospital in the Bulgarian capital, all when at her most vulnerable. At this point, could the momentary intrusion of a strange American man with a notebook possibly faze her?

12   Medical tourism can best be defined as cross-border travel for the primary purpose of securing treatment. The term may suggest carefree holidaymakers, but like the Libyan knee patient, many medical tourists are engaged in a uniquely modern form of rebellion, asserting an individual's independence from the persistence of political geography.

For a long time, such "patients with passports"—as Harvard Law Professor I. Glenn Cohen called them in the title of his recent book on the legal and ethical dynamics of medical tourism—were only the unfavorably situated. They were wealthy patients stuck in underdeveloped countries, those unable to afford complex procedures where they live and desperate enough to hunt down a bargain, and patients suffering from peculiar maladies in places without the right specialists. Indeed, the most famous classical examples—Gulf sheiks flying to the Mayo Clinic on a private jet, or North Americans heading south for inexpensive breast implants—share in-extremis attributes, either for care that is an absolute necessity or pure luxury. In short, people traveled for the same reasons tourists always have: to find what they are unable to get at home.

For medical tourists coming to the United States, that tends to be access to care. For American medical tourists heading elsewhere, it is usually lower costs. After all, the same system that produced the Mayo Clinic—and enough doctors, specialized equipment and empty beds to welcome the world's well-heeled walk-in patients—leaves many local residents unable to afford even basic procedures. A 2014 study from the Commonwealth Fund concluded that American health care was both more expensive and less effective than that of ten

other similarly industrialized western countries, economics
that trickle down to individual patients. The National Center
for Policy Analysis in 2007 estimated one with insurance could
expect to pay $90,000 for a heart bypass in the United States,
but only about $20,000 if traveling to Singapore, $12,000
in Thailand, and $10,000 in India. One of the 30 million
Americans without medical insurance could expect to pay more
than $200,000 for the procedure at a local hospital.

No institution has pursued opportunity in medical tourism
like Bumrungrad International Hospital, in Bangkok, Thailand.
First opened in 1980 with 200 beds, it has expanded to several
times that, claiming to serve 1.1 million patients annually, about
half of them from abroad. For those from countries more developed than Thailand, Bumrungrad is a bargain. For those from
countries less developed, Bumrungrad offers access to specialized expertise or equipment unavailable at home. In other cases,
Thai doctors will perform specific procedures—most notably,
sexual reassignment surgery—that law or custom preclude
elsewhere. Bumrungrad now has thirty different specialized
centers under its roof, but the hospital's marketing materials
tend to emphasize non-medical capacities there, such as the two
hotels it operates and a permanent visa-processing center that
the Thai Home Ministry has set up on-site to facilitate exten-
sions for patients. The hospital employs 109 interpreters, which
it says covers the range of languages spoken by patients representing 190 countries. (Appropriately enough, "Bumrungrad"
doesn't mean anything in any known tongue, although it is more
or less pronounceable in most of them.) In 2004, based on the
success of Bumrungrad and many like-minded Thai hospitals

14 that have followed it, the government launched a marketing campaign branding Thailand the "Medical Hub of Asia."

But despite Thailand's claim, the impression that medicine revolves around any particular hospital or country has been unmasked as the type of fiction devised by investment-promotion authorities and indulged by their ad agencies eager to promote someplace as "the medical capital of the world." Due to developments as seemingly banal as the ability to quickly move high-resolution X-ray images as email attachments, patients can travel for care anywhere, even to hospitals that don't have their own hotels connected by walkway.

Across the world, globalization has transformed the pursuit of better health outcomes. Linking high-speed fiber optic networks via undersea cable has made possible the field known as telemedicine, in which the internet is used to facilitate long-distance care through real-time monitoring of patients. tThe integration of once geographically bounded labor markets has led doctors to outsource support tasks, like the reading of X-rays, to countries where they can be completed at lower costs. (Many X-rays taken in American clinics are viewed by Indian radiologists.) In the pharmaceutical industry, multinational corporations have proven able to simultaneously exploit advanced economies' research capacity and legal systems to support innovation, and developing countries' lower manufacturing costs to bring the resultant products cheaply to market.

But more than other high-skilled services (like finance and law), most medical talent and infrastructure remain stubbornly grounded in place. When it comes to medical procedures, there is only so much marketers can do to shuttle goods or facilitate the delivery of services. Medical tourism has never demanded much beyond air travel and payments across currencies. Sometimes, as in the plentiful cases of Americans driving across the Mexican border and paying doctors and dentists in dollars, it requires neither.

In the years since Bumrungrad opened, medical tourism has become a dizzyingly multidirectional affair. While one can easily rationalize how Brazil found so much of its national identity tied up in a role as a provider of plastic surgery, many of the grooved routes of medical tourism don't display a self-evident logic. Emiratis fly to South Korea for organ transplants. Canadians travel to Costa Rica for checkups. Yemenis with heart disease often end up in India. Cypriots requiring bone-marrow transplants go to Israel. Each pairing seems to be conjured from a game of Risk, which in its way makes sense, because the unique risk management involved in medical care has bonded countries that have never had particularly deep trade links, migration flows, or military or diplomatic ties.

The logic that sustains the routes of medical tourism has less to do with the connections between countries than the gaps between them. Medical tourism requires seeing national differences as inefficiencies that can be exploited. Within Europe, where neighboring countries share cultural attributes and increasingly the same economic policies, medical systems often came to define the nation-state in the process of shedding its other totems of national identity. (A 2013 survey in the United Kingdom ranked its National Health Service the institution that made people proudest to be British, ahead of the monarchy and the BBC.)

The integration that has remade Europe in the twentieth century—a common currency, elimination of travel restrictions, and a deregulated airspace that has permitted low-cost carriers to take flight—has remapped the region's medical geography. Once far-off capitals are often now no farther or pricier to get to than taking a half-day's drive. Europeans increasingly conditioned to hopscotch the continent for leisure are finding it just as practical to do so in search of better, cheaper, or more readily available health-care services. For Europeans, political and logistical changes have conspired to make medical tourism a quotidian, even humdrum, practice.

But those who engage in it quickly learn that they will have to do so without the security of a transnational safety net. In attempting to stitch together the first strands of one, the European Union has illustrated the difficulty of coming up with any sort of health-care policy that applies equally across borders. To American eyes, the machinations that have taken place in Brussels evoke what it might be like to observe a Congress trying to simultaneously negotiate an interlocking health-care reform bill and trade pact, all under the watchful eye of a Supreme Court that has determined that core constitutional rights and freedoms are at stake. (Imagine further that the central question of health-care reform was whether Germans should pay for its citizens to use Greek hospitals by traversing the same open borders that permit Syrian refugees to settle freely in Europe.) Is it possible to develop a system that allows citizens to take advantage of the benefits they have been promised by their public and private insurers all while exercising their right to travel and trade freely?

Medical tourists have come to represent a small but revealing new tranche of the worldwide middle class, empowered to arbitrage inefficiencies created where a previous era's institutions of political economy—namely insurance companies and national regulatory régimes—had failed to keep up with a new era's interconnectedness. In an increasingly globalized world, national governments may be losing control over flows of money and information, but they are still responsible for health care. Medical tourism exists only because the great triumph of liberal government in the twentieth century and the neoliberal project of free movement for people and capital have proven fundamentally irreconcilable. What happens when all the other national boundaries fall and the most salient difference between neighboring countries is in their health-care systems?

I had ended up in Eastern Europe because a sequence of political transformations had dramatically accelerated the pace of that reckoning. In the 1990s, centrally planned medical systems in former Soviet Bloc nations were exposed to domestic market forces, introducing competition for patients into a health economy that had previously known no notion of profit. Just as they were beginning to calibrate a post-communist balance between the competing interests of the marketplace and the welfare state, the countries of Eastern Europe sought entry to the European Union. In so doing, they opened themselves—their borders, their banks, their operating theatres—to any European who wanted to access them.

Almost instantaneously Eastern European countries found themselves inevitably part of what the Canadian health

18   researcher Ronald Labonté has described as a worldwide "gold
      rush of primarily private, but also some public, providers in
      low- and middle-income countries attempting to capitalize on
      what they perceive to be an unfilled demand from the wealthier
      and demographically aging North." My reporting in Hungary
      and Bulgaria is an attempt to trace the opening of one sluice
      in this gold rush, and its effect on the people and institutions
      it touches. Is medical tourism destabilizing one of the last
      remaining pillars of the welfare state or reinforcing it?

      Many critics of medical tourism cast its existence along
      familiar lines of global inequality, with the implication that it
      is impossible to reconcile a health-care system that profits from
      serving foreigners and one that succeeds in serving the local
      community's needs. In Tokuda Hospital Sofia's orthopedics
      wing, that conundrum was given a face. What did the presence
      of a Libyan woman in a Bulgarian hospital bed mean for a Sofia
      resident with knee problems? And could Libya ever develop a
      modern health-care system if all the local patients who had a
      way of financing their care took their problems—and their
      money—elsewhere?

      It was easy to caricature medical tourists as the world's
      haves taking medicine from the mouth of its have-nots, but
      the woman before me certainly did not project an air of entitle-
      ment. I was reminded of the many levels of dislocation involved
      whenever an individual decided not to let her ability to imag-
      ine a healthier self be constrained by the boundaries of her
      home nation.

Orbán's Dentist

Among the regular cast of characters who populate the pages of Hungary's newspapers and magazines, the one whose fame is hardest to understand in a country long proud of its disproportionate achievement in the field of Olympic medals and Nobel prizes may be the man usually identified simply as the prime minister's dentist.

Béla Bátorfi's rise to fame can be traced to the 2010 return of the conservative Fidesz party after eight years of Socialist Party dominance. Bátorfi, then forty-one years old, had a thriving practice in a posh residential corner of Buda with a clientele that included an impressive slice of the Budapest political elite. Among his longtime clients was the new prime minister, Viktor Orbán, who had been his patient for almost twenty years. Orbán developed a reputation for ruthlessly punishing opponents and rewarding supporters, naming Fidesz loyalists to posts in the central bank and office of the chief prosecutor—departments

20   that had been previously immune to partisan politics. "'Orbán
is putting his people everywhere,' is a constant lament in
Budapest," the *Economist* itself lamented early in his term. Even
the man who tended to the first family's teeth stood to benefit.

Bátorfi is indeed a specialist in oral surgery, with a dental degree from his country's most celebrated medical college,
Semmelweis University, and a masters from the University of
Münster in Germany. But when his name appears in Hungarian
newspapers it is rarely in direct connection to his proficiency
with a drill or scalpel. Most frequently, Bátorfi is covered as a
subject of political intrigue. When, in his second year in office,
Orbán invited dental businesses to bid for a series of government tenders, Bátorfi entered and ultimately won everything for
which he appeared to be eligible. ("It is possible to get the money
through a complex application, but inevitably Viktor Orbán's
dentist's company will be awarded the billion forints," the news
website Origo had predicted before one such grant process was
complete.) Over the first four years of Orbán's administration, 3 billion forints in contracts and state aid (equal to roughly
10 million dollars) have flowed from the federal government of
Hungary to a congeries of companies and trade associations
under Bátorfi's influence. "Bátorfi has been Orbán's dentist since
1992," László Szűcs, a Bátorfi adviser, told the news magazine *Heti
Világgazdaság,* defending his client's right to bid for government
tenders that he would eventually win. "Why wouldn't he enter
into a competition when any other business could compete?"

That sense of infinite possibility now infuses nearly everything Bátorfi does. He also chairs his own eponymous athletic
club, based in the northeastern city of Eger, and presides over the

Budapest Ironman competition as president of the Hungarian Triathlon Union. "He is expanding into the entertainment business, and could open a famous club in Eger with municipal or state assistance, or take part in a planned real-estate development," *Heti Világgazdaság* reported in the summer of 2014.

The patients responsible for the wealth amassed by the Bátorfi Dental Implant Clinic, however, were unlikely to have ever read about any of its proprietor's political, sporting, or entrepreneurial exploits. Instead, they knew him only as the studious dentist with an unusually high number of advertisements in London media. "The proof of his work and competence are the more than 35,000 patients he has treated. Dr. Bátorfi is honest and always ready to share his knowledge and expertise with his patients," declared an ad that Bátorfi placed in *The Times* to promote a clinic that he had branded the British-Hungarian Medical Service. "What he lacked in bedside manner he made up for with efficiency," a travel writer for the *Telegraph* wrote about a series of 2007 visits to Budapest for implant surgery, noting that by his second visit Bátorfi's "communication skills had not progressed much beyond the 'open now' and 'close now' level, and his fast fingers seemed fatter than before."

Unlike Orbán, Bátorfi's patients from abroad typically saw the clinic's self-described master implantologist only once or twice, if ever. Much as luck had once placed a promising young parliamentarian into his dental chair years before he would make good in politics, a fortuitous connection had introduced Bátorfi to the practice of medical tourism years before the phrase meant much of anything to anyone.

In 2000, a Hungarian based in England had approached Bátorfi with a proposal. If he could persuade Brits to take advantage of cheap and available Hungarian dental work, would the dentist share with him a cut of the new business?

Bátorfi got a license to practice in the UK and rented an office in London. To Bátorfi's surprise, the patients started coming, adventurous types willing to confront the unfamiliar in search of prices that—even with all travel expenses included—typically fell below half of what they might pay in Bristol or Belfast. "In the beginning, that an English dentist would recommend a Hungarian dentist was unbelievable," Bátorfi marvels today.

He was nimble enough to reorient his practice to satisfy the new business. Recognizing that foreign customers would be most likely to travel for expensive treatments where they could realize the greatest savings, Bátorfi chose to pursue his masters in implantology, which includes some of oral surgery's most complex procedures. Back in Budapest, he began setting his prices in British pounds and offering free chauffeur pickup at the airport. Bátorfi spent $150,000 per year on marketing, in addition to other extravagant gestures. About a decade ago, Bátorfi spent approximately $200,000 to acquire four pieces of equipment that László Szűcs calls "the Rolls-Royce of dental chairs." Szűcs claims that there are only four other existing versions of the same model, manufactured by the Japanese company Morita: one owned by Russian President Vladimir Putin, one by German Chancellor Angela Merkel, and two by a private Swedish clinic.

Since then, Bátorfi—who appears year-round with a tan that gives the impression that he has uncovered a secret yacht passage from the Danube to the Mediterranean—has become

the perfectly bronzed face of one of the most unexpectedly shim-
mering sectors of Hungary's post-communist economy. Between
2000 and 2008, the number of per-capita dentists in Hungary
increased by 56 percent. Many of them were eager to follow
Bátorfi into the increasingly well-defined sphere known as medical tourism, in which patients travel to another country with
the primary purpose of securing treatment. Hungary has more
dentists per head of population than any other country, according to London journalist David Hancock, who in 2006 wrote a
guide for British patients called *The Complete Medical Tourist.*
"And since the country joined the European Union their fellow
Europeans have had plenty to smile about, too, because prices are
considerably cheaper there than in neighboring countries like
Austria and Germany," Hancock wrote. "No wonder Hungarians
smile a lot!"

Not everyone was smiling about Hungarian dentistry's international profile. The country had struggled since the end of its
communist era to deliver quality health coverage within a market economy to all its citizens. To those, particularly within
rural areas, the fact that the most lucrative part of Hungarian
health care was a gaudily extravagant sector that existed largely
to serve foreigners' vanities appeared to be a failure of government, a moral abomination.

By the time Orbán became prime minister, medical tourism had become widely accepted by policymakers as unique
tool for economic development. Its promise was almost magi-
cal: tourism for countries that had not been gifted with beaches
or mountains, or had lacked the good sense millennia ago to

24   preserve their abandoned stone structures for future sightsee-
ing purposes.

When his patient and friend became head of government,
Bátorfi's language began to shift from speaking of his own
five-chair dental clinic as the dominant center of commerce to
talking about his country of 10 million as a whole. He began to
contemplate the ways that medical tourism had converted his
own business from a diverse family-oriented dental practice
to a high-value oral-surgery outfit, and whether the dominant
market position he had assumed could be extrapolated into
a type of national comparative advantage. A 2010 study by the
country's central tax bureau estimated that the 60,000 dental
tourists who traveled to Hungary each year generated 65 billion forints (about $250 million) in revenue for dentists, with
another 13 billion forints or $5 million in ancillary spending on
hotels and restaurants. The sector had survived the recession,
and business showed little sign of slowing. After all, the peculiar
dynamics that brought people to Bátorfi's London clinic for consultations and onward to Budapest for surgery—a British health
system that made certain types of medical care scarce, or costly,
or both—weren't likely to yield anytime soon. "There are few
things in which Hungary is in a leading position, and dental tourism is the one," he says.

When the British dental profession started to push back
at the Hungarian invasion of its home turf, it started with
Bátorfi himself. In 2011, he was informed that the British Dental
Association had suspended his license to practice dentistry
in the United Kingdom for one year. All the details suggested
a process driven by the desire to make an example of him, or

possibly even a personal vendetta. Charges of malpractice were
based on the testimony of a patient who had, five years earlier,
traveled to Budapest for implant surgery and were sketchy about
specifying actual damages. (Bátorfi was alleged to have given
insufficient advance information about the treatment plan and,
after the patient expressed dissatisfaction with the procedure,
had not responded to follow-up queries about options for cor-
rective treatment.)

A month later, after an appeal, the suspension was
rescinded, but not before the prime minister's dentist had been
elevated into a national symbol of Hungary's ability to put
wealthier countries on the defensive.

That year, Hungary's Medical Tourism Office, which Bátorfi as
director operates as his vehicle for designing a national strategy,
organized a dental tourism conference in Budapest, at which
Orbán's government signed a cooperation agreement with the
sector and announced its first billion-forint grant. "A worthy
and good investment," Orbán said there. The financial commitment was a bet that medical tourism was more than a fad—that
what had very quickly shown Hungary to be effective at luring travelers to seek medical care there wasn't just the consequence of a few talented dentists emerging at the right time, or
of Bátorfi's preternatural instinct for entrepreneurialism. Had
Hungary made itself good at something that would last?

After officially winning the public contract to determine
how that "worthy and good investment" would be spent, Bátorfi
turned to yet another one of his patients for help. László Szűcs
was a communications consultant based in Budapest whom

26   Bátorfi had informally asked for marketing advice in between visits to the dental chair for years, before asking him to serve as CEO of the Medical Tourism Office. When Bátorfi had first put Szűcs on his payroll, in 2009, Szűcs was in Napa Valley, working on a short documentary about Croatian-American winemaker Mike Grgich, whose Chateau Montelena Chardonnay famously won the 1976 Judgment of Paris competition, establishing California wines as a formidable product with a distinct identity in the global marketplace. Szűcs and Miklos Rózsa, a business consultant whom Bátorfi was able to pay with European Union funds acquired through Orbán's government, began thinking about their product in similar terms.

"Our aim is," Rózsa says, "'in Switzerland, you get chocolates and watches. In Hungary, you get dentistry.'"

Bismarck and Beveridge

For millennia, the most ambitious programs in medical treatment could be understood as a quest for natural resources.

Tubercular patients hunted altitudes that would immerse them in thin air. Those with sore joints sought to soak in thermal waters where they gurgled from the earth. Some popular tourist destinations—Taos, St. Moritz, Baden-Baden—began as idyllic refuges for the ill.

In the late eighteenth century, when the discovery of vaccines heralded the arrival of modern medicine, those topographical advantages began to give way. Instead, deft surgeons and skilled pharmacists began to cluster in places where they would have access to the increasingly specialized tools or chemical compounds necessary for their crafts, and the infrastructure to support the work they did. In the nineteenth century, the public hospital became the dominant site for managing medical care, displacing the fieldwork of religious institutions. By

28   the twentieth century, scientific advances meant that medicine
        could actually improve a patient's health as opposed to merely
        placating the ill and containing the spread of disease. "It has
        often been said that it was not until this century that the average
        patient who consulted the average doctor was likely to derive
        benefit from the encounter," British health economist Brian
        Abel-Smith observed in 1976.

        Medicine became integral to bettering society, and thus
        a matter for policy makers. In its Universal Declaration of
        Human Rights, the United Nations in 1948 decreed, "Everyone
        has the right to a standard of living adequate for the health and
        well-being of himself and of his family, including food, cloth-
        ing, housing and medical care and necessary social services."
        The declaration offered the fifty-eight countries who were
        then members no further guidance about what "medical care"
        entails and who would have the responsibility of providing it.

        In the 1880s, Germany's Otto von Bismarck had begun
        experimenting with the idea that the state could serve as a bro-
        ker between the sick, the people who could help them, and the
        institutions that could afford to pay for that care. Attempting
        to staunch the flow of Germans to North America in search
        of greater economic opportunity, Bismarck promised public
        insurance to his country's workers. His chosen mechanism for
        extending that coverage was indirect, relying on a program of
        public reimbursements to largely private medical providers
        augmented with individually acquired insurance plans.

        A half-century later, the United Kingdom eschewed
        Bismarck's decentralized approach. A 1942 report titled *Social
        Insurance and Allied Services* chaired by economist and social

reformer William Beveridge—later known as the *Beveridge Report*, the blueprint for the modern British welfare state—had asserted that "restoration of a sick person to health is a duty of the State and the sick person." But when Beveridge's recommendations were turned into policy the burden fell largely on the state. In 1946, Britain chartered the National Health Service, which unified the country's entire health infrastructure and all its personnel within one organization. Under this so-called single-payer system, the federal government both controlled the financing and delivery of all medicine to citizens, using tax revenues to ensure that treatment was free at the time of care.

The Bismarck system and the Beveridge system became the dominant models worldwide for countries seeking an answer to the question: How does a government protect its citizens against the risk of injury and illness, and preside over their inevitable decline with age? In 1978, the World Health Organization, which had embraced the slogan "Health for All," hosted a conference for health ministers to articulate that as an ostensibly attainable goal. "Governments have a responsibility for the health of their people which can be fulfilled only by the provision of adequate health and social measures," asserted the Alma Ata Declaration adopted by 134 countries. (The Kazakh city where the declaration was produced is now known as Almaty.) "A main social target of governments, international organizations and the whole world community in the coming decades should be the attainment by all peoples of the world by the year 2000 of a level of health that will permit them to lead a socially and economically productive life."

30   The year 2000 came and went, and today approximately sixty countries have accomplished what could be considered universal health care for their citizenries. (The definition, and even the distinction between "universal health care" and "universal coverage," is highly contested among experts.) Other countries, such as the United States, have developed systems that give government regulators a major role in bending medical economics toward desired policy outcomes, even as they fall short of providing health care to all citizens. (The United States has been an exception by relying on a largely private model in which most insurance is supplied by companies to employees.)

Each country's health policies have developed according to its peculiar circumstances. National systems retain traces of the labor economies from which they emerged—whether designed to serve a nation of shopkeepers, farmers, or factory workers—and a citizenry's acceptance of higher taxes in exchange for services. Cultural and social dynamics affected whether individual health was treated as a private or public responsibility, if this was manifest in a constitutional guarantee, and how its existing legal framework weighed those competing interests. The relative logic of a scheme demonstrates whether a country conceived a holistic system at once—and had a strong enough central government to implement it—or reflected the series of incremental adjustments, tweaks, and negotiations often compelled by a divided political structure.

Even when considered in the abstract, health-care reform has long been a whack-a-mole game for policy makers. Reduce prices, and you often diminish supply, as doctors earn less per procedure. Expanding access to care increases costs across the system. Making the latest scientific breakthroughs available to as many people as possible often requires discouraging the innovation that makes them possible. Improving the quality of specialty care can make it prohibitively expensive, or too scarce to be accessible. Every approach to health-care reform means, effectively, choosing to accept one dysfunction to avoid another. Taiwan has accomplished universal coverage with low premiums, but suffers from doctor shortages in part because of the long hours and low pay associated with their jobs. The United States has created conditions that enable rarified specialists to thrive even if most citizens can't access their care.

Whether a streamlined piece of exquisite social engineering like Taiwan's single-payer program or a sprawling jerry-rigged contraption like the American régime, a national health-care system is as distinctive a creative product as the modern nation-state has yet generated. Political scientists speculate that shared patterns of industrialization and the globalization of political knowledge are leading to increasingly common policy prescriptions, a model they call convergence theory. But medicine appears relatively immune to the trend. Even if reforms and innovations are indeed leading to a convergence of once-distinct models—"towards the Bev-marck or Bis-eridge model," as World Health Organization financing-policy coordinator Joseph Kutzin has put it—national health systems are still marked by pronounced idiosyncrasies.

Even neighboring countries with otherwise comparable populations and natural resources can maintain radically different economies around health care. Since Canada overhauled its health-care regulations in 1984, its system and that of its

32   only neighbor have continued to diverge. In the United States, where a lack of price controls has historically made medicine incredibly lucrative, many individual doctors pursue narrow specialties. Scarcity is rarely a concern for patients, but price almost always is. (Reforms under the Affordable Care Act push the United States toward the Bismarck model, although with some significant differences that make American health care still much more expensive.) Canada, in which the federal government runs a single-payer system along the Beveridge model, has produced the inverse. Canadians seeking even basic care face long waits for appointments, but never worry about cost.

Multinational currency unions, border agreements, defense pacts, and transcontinental free-trade zones have gradually shrunken many of the twentieth century's defining markers of the nation-state. It is easy to imagine a day where an individual who steps over the world's longest unguarded border experiences no political or economic change whatsoever, unless she happens to damage her knee with that step. On one side, she would fall into a web of government-owned hospitals where all services are funded by the federal budget. On the other, she would confront an array of largely private clinics and hospitals whose work was supported by a mixture of public reimbursements and individually held insurance plans. Even adjacent countries with comparably structured systems for insurance like France and Belgium are not designed to offer any interoperability between them.

In that cozy fit of unique health systems and national borders, medical tourism amounts to playing in the margins. The

disconnect between geographic proximity and regulatory distance represents an opportunity for arbitrage that is as much a
feature of globalization as the other links that make possible the
trans-border flow of capital and labor. The only limits are often
ingenuity and patience. Laws typically do not forbid individuals from traveling in search of better health outcomes. People
and money can move freely across national boundaries, but the
safeguards that national governments have imposed to protect their citizens from the unpredictable—safety-net insurance, consumer protections, the ability to sue for malpractice
claims—usually do not.

As health care becomes a more important component of
national economies—it is now the fastest growing sector of the
United States—it has become difficult to balance concerns for
the local population with an appetite for international competitiveness. Patent and trademark laws are meant to protect intel-
lectual property like pharmaceutical drugs, but their reliance on
national legal codes looks increasingly outdated in an era when
the fruits of that discovery can move effortlessly across borders.
Yet even as countries work to synchronize intellectual-property
laws, there are no efforts to homogenize national health systems. Not even the most ambitious utopian thinker or worldly
philanthropist imagines a single global standard for health-care
delivery. (Within the United States it is hard enough to lower
the barriers separating states' insurance markets.)

Because each imperfect system is imperfect in its own way,
almost inevitably any two systems will reveal asymmetries as
their economies integrate in other spheres. In 1994, Canada
and the United States (along with Mexico) adopted the North

34   American Free Trade Agreement, which removed tariffs and import quotes to establish a common market for most goods and services. The agreement, which took effect in 1994, specifically singled out "law enforcement, correctional services, income security or insurance, social security or insurance, social welfare, public education, public training, health, and child care" as service sectors exempt from its requirements to relax non-tariff barriers to trade, such as import licenses and local-content requirements. All are essentially functions in which government regulation can be understood to support a public-policy objective rather than purely a private profit motive. Most remained by their nature stubbornly immune to the globalizing pressures of a newly connected world. No nation, after all, is competing for another's prisoners.

That classification has had the impact of creating separate rules for economies of medical goods and medical services. While it remains illegal for Americans to "re-import" cheaper drugs from Canada, where prices are much lower because of looser intellectual-property rules governing pharmaceutical copyright, nothing stops sick Canadians from crossing the border to make an appointment with American specialists. Because the economics of medicine are shaped by regulations at the place of delivery, those doctors have no interest in relocating their practices to be closer to consumers, the way a manufacturer of automobiles might.

The burden of navigating this world of globalized medicine falls disproportionately on individual consumers. It is up to them to discover and exploit new discontinuities like gaps between supply and demand, and, perhaps most important, the imparity in price and quality of care. Corporations and governments are forced to respond and adjust, but the supply of medical tourists seems to shift more readily than potential destinations are able to adjust to the changes. Countries that find themselves newly wealthy have learned that investments in tourist infrastructure can quickly recast them as destinations for leisure or convention travelers but do little to address the underlying shortcomings of their medical systems. In fact, South Korea has established its position in the medical-tourism economy in part by catering specifically to the inability of wealthy Persian Gulf states to serve their own citizens' organ-transplant needs. The Emirati government, for example, is rich enough to often fully reimburse citizens when they travel overseas for coverage, but it has historically been unable to marshal those resources to assemble a labor force prepared to handle complex specialty procedures. Dubai had the world's tallest building before it had a single organ-transplant hospital. (The Emirates' first opened in 2014.)

Even as European integration has had a flattening effect on mobility within the continent, the idiosyncrasies of local medical economies remain too deeply rooted in place to shift quickly. Conditions are set above all by local regulatory and financing régimes, the product of national political conditions that make ongoing reform unlikely. Given the arduous pace of medical education, particularly for unusual specialties, health-care capacity often operates on a generation-long delay; today's doctors selected their skills decades ago. In Hungary, vestiges of Prussian education and Soviet politics mix to give the country a supply of highly qualified dentists unable to maximize their earning potential with local patients alone.

36   Hungary's emergence as Europe's dental chair is a story of how quickly a country can claim a comparative advantage, can brand itself as a destination for a particular set of services, and how potentially durable that market position can be. Medicine may be the rare area of human endeavor where place matters more than it did one or two hundred years ago. One country's comparative advantages over another can last a generation. So can its deficiencies.

Torn Curtain

On August 30, 1987, a fifty-four-year-old dentist named László Szilágyi, along with his wife Zsuzsanna and their small son, set out from Budapest and drove just about as far to the northwest as was possible before running into the highly militarized border that had been erected to keep Hungarians like them from escaping into Austria. All they knew was that two mornings later, Szilágyi would have to report to a dental chair in a town called Sopron. "We didn't know where we'd sleep," recalls Pai Szilágyi, László's son, "but we knew when my father had to be at work."

Both of the adult Szilágyis were dentists, and for years they had been following the narrow path of opportunity afforded to ambitious or restless doctors in communist Hungary. Unlike other Eastern European countries, which treated dentists as specialized doctors, the Hungarian medical sector had considered it as a separate profession. (At the time, the field was often

38   known as stomatology.) For a while, this mattered most in medical schools, where dentists (like pharmacists) followed an alto-
gether different path of study from those seeking to be licensed
as physicians. When the country took its first fitful steps toward
permitting small-scale private enterprises, doctors weren't eligible to participate, but dentists could.

While living in eastern Hungary, just miles from Ukraine,
László Szilágyi had become proprietor of one of the country's
earliest private dental clinics. When offered the opportunity
to join another—the larger Dental Coop, which had opened in
1984 to serve the Budapest elite—Szilágyi packed his dental
equipment, along with the rest of his family's possessions, into
two trucks and pointed them toward the capital. Now barely a
year and a half after that, the Szilágyis were moving again, for
a city of barely 50,000 that László knew only from its rich past.

Szilágyi arrived for duty at the Pannonia Hotel, one of the
first dentists hired to staff a clinic that had opened six months
earlier. The Pannonia Hotel had been in existence since 1893,
but before that an inn called the Golden Bull had sat at the same
location for centuries. Its history, punctuated by regular fires,
encapsulated Sopron's shifting appeal to out-of-town visitors. (Pannonia was the name the Romans who settled the area
gave to the part of their empire now known as trans-Danubia.)
Tucked in the country's northwest corner near both Austria
and Czechoslovakia, Sopron had traded custody between
crowns and countries and managed to maintain layered archi-
tectural traces of each period in an intact town center that was
an appealing destination for domestic tourists. During the
Cold War, when the property was assumed by the state-owned

Hungar Hotels chain, the Pannonia often served as a way-station for East German holidaymakers en route to Hungary's scenic Lake Balaton for their summer vacations.

The fact that a dental clinic had set up shop on the hotel's first floor was an early indicator of an unusually promising future for Sopron. The stretch of the Iron Curtain separating Hungary from its neighbors—where once Hungarian rail operators locked car doors as their trains briefly passed through Austrian territory—was growing increasingly porous over the course of the 1980s. Vienna residents willing to transverse the well-fortified border were able to choose from twenty dentists trained to Prussian standards but stuck working at Soviet prices. "That's the key driver of why Austrians come to Hungary, because everything is cheaper," says Tamás Karakai, CEO of Sopron's Wabi Beauty Center. "We use the same equipment, but the wages and energy are much lower in Hungary."

On August 19, 1989, Sopron was the site of the Pan-European Picnic, planned by Hungarian dissidents as an occasion for their fellow citizens to meet their Austrian neighbors. In the afternoon's social détente, Hungarian authorities spied an elegant solution to a refugee crisis roiling within their borders, with East Germans who had come to Hungary for their summer vacations unwilling to return to their homes. As thousands of local residents mingled in the no-man's land between the two countries, hundreds of East Germans were directed toward an intentionally unguarded wooden gate, effectively invited to make their way to West Germany through Austria. The episode, which concluded with little drama and Moscow's tacit acceptance, presaged the Berlin Wall's collapse months

40   later. When Germany completed the process of reunification the following year, Chancellor Helmut Kohl reflected that it was in Sopron where "the first stone was knocked out of the wall."

The Szilágyis had been active in organizing the picnic, and found themselves among the first in Sopron to fully realize the opportunity that would accompany the geopolitical shifts that would follow. With the boundary between Western and Eastern Europe reduced to just another humdrum border crossing, Sopron became effectively a Vienna exurb—less than one hour, by train or car, from the city center—with a wide array of dental services at a fraction of the cost. "You could see what was coming in the early 1990s," says Pai Szilágyi. "You couldn't move on the streets of Sopron because there were so many Austrians."

Soon, Sopron became known across Central Europe as much for the dentists' clinics that were popping up between the baroque structures and the Roman ruins as for those monuments themselves. (A smaller Hungarian town, Mosonmagyaróvár, farther from the Austrian border but with better highway connections, found itself even better positioned to receive patients from Vienna.) "The demand was growing much, much faster than the supply, so we did not need marketing," says László Szilágyi.

The Szilágyis worked seven days a week, with a half-day on Sunday to give the family enough time for dinner together, and learned German along the way. They performed a variety of dental services—inlays, fillings, implants, crowns—but refused to do purely cosmetic work, which László Szilágyi called "a question of medical ethics." The clinic had six dentists staffing four patient chairs, along with a large operating room and a smaller one for a technician. It became an immensely profitable practice.

As Hungary abandoned its communist system for free-market capitalism, the government began selling off many of its assets, including its state-run hotels. The Szilágyis had never shown interest in entering the hospitality sector, but in an increasingly crowded marketplace in Sopron their dental practice's brand—reinforced through referrals and word-of-mouth—was tied up in its unique location. "They knew him as the dentist in the Pannonia Hotel," Pai Szilágyi says of his father. At a government auction in 1992, the family won the bid to secure a fifteen-year loan to purchase the sixty-two-room property, and they became hoteliers.

The Szilágyis soon discovered that the hotel business was generating new dental patients, not the other way around, as they had initially expected. Starting in 1995, they tried rebranding the facility as the Pannonia Medical Hotel, but eventually dropped the label after it became evident it wasn't doing much to improve occupancy rates. Most of the dental clinic's patients lived within range of an easy cross-border day trip. (A commitment to join the Best Western chain proved more durable than the rebranding.) Zsuszanna cut her dental shifts in half, spending the rest of the week managing the hotel. "We are still dentists," says László Szilágyi. "We never paid enough attention to the hotel. It was always like a hobby."

Sopron's entire hospitality sector was similarly distracted by the city's new fascination with teeth. In 1996, the general manager of the Pannonia's restaurant left his job and—despite having no medical background—opened his own dental clinic

42   around the corner from the hotel. By the turn of the century, Sopron had become the one city in this pastry-mad country where it was easier to find someone skilled in fixing cavities than a vendor of the sweets liable to provoke them.

The dental profession was itself in flux. In 1995, as part of an effort to cut its budget, Hungary had privatized dental operations in state and local hospitals nationwide. While the country has a nationalized health-care system, few Hungarians carry extra insurance, and so typically pay for dental care with cash. Dentists saw their turn to thrive outside the single-payer framework, and in the three years that followed the country gained 1,371 private dental facilities. Many recognized the value of catering to international patients, as did those looking to enter the profession anew. The number of foreign students in dental programs at Hungary's four medical universities grew in the years that followed, with much of that increase coming from students choosing to receive their training in either the English or German language rather than Hungarian. (By 2005, all four of the schools offered English-language programs.)

In 2004, Hungary entered the European Union, beginning the process of obliterating land and air crossings as part of the Schengen migration agreement that allowed passport-free travel within the continent. At the same time that travel within Europe became freer, it also grew cheaper. Deregulation of the continent's airspace opened up the travel marketplace, under-mining many national carriers that had had effective monop-olies at their home airports and allowing new competitors to enter with lower fares. The arrival of low-cost carriers, par-ticularly the Budapest-based Wizz Air, redrew the catchment

area around Hungarian dentists. A few hours' drive from the
border towns of Sopron and Mosonmagyaróvár encompassed
all of Austria and population centers in Germany and Italy. A
few hours' flight from Ferihegy Airport covered everything from
Dublin to Moscow and the entire Mediterranean Basin.

The Bátorfi Dental Implant Clinic was positioned to benefit. At
the time Béla Bátorfi had first been approached by his London
contact proposing that they work together, in 2000, there was
only a single Budapest dentistry that served primarily foreign patients. Many of them were Hungarians living overseas
or people of Hungarian descent (including some Hungarian-
Americans) who sought to combine dental treatment with other
scheduled trips. For a few years, Bátorfi had the overseas market to himself, but almost immediately after Wizz Air's launch
Bátorfi had familiar competition. Attila Kaman, based nearby
in Buda, reoriented his clinic along similar lines after studying
Bátorfi's, aggressively advertising on English and Irish televi-
sion and radio, eventually experimenting with online campaigns, as well. "He was my friend, asked everything about my
business, and then copied it," Bátorfi tells me.

   They were not alone. Malev Air Tours, affiliated with
Hungary's now-defunct flag carrier, began offering a dental
examination as part of its tour packages, the same way it might
include an admission ticket to the zoo. "It's nothing expensive,
just a cheap extra—you always put in an extra to hide the cost,"
says Peter Takács, the tour company's managing director. "With
this solution you can say 'we are the cheapest option' because
no one else offers it." Dentists who ran Budapest offices with

44   traditional community-oriented practices—serving a combination of nearby families and expatriates—began to adjust away from the high-volume work of cleanings and fillings and toward the more lucrative procedures that people might find worth traveling for. "They let the local patients go," says dentist Zoltán Szakács. Eventually, according to one estimate by academic researchers, around 80 percent of dentists in the Transdanubia region opened offices in Budapest.

Clinics found the English and Irish markets so satisfied by Budapest operations that they started looking for other European countries where they could build a patient base. The Apollonia Dental Center opened in 2007 and began to focus its marketing efforts on France, where an implant and crown procedure that a Budapest clinic could offer for 800 euros was priced at 1,700 euros. "The dental hygiene of French people is worse," says chief operating officer Brigitta Fehér, "so their need is bigger than the Italians." Eventually the clinic hired two French-speaking coordinators to arrange consultations at a Parisian X-ray center and prepare patients for a potentially disorienting experience abroad. "The attitude of French patients is a little bit surprised how well developed Hungary is," says Fehér. "They have a prejudice about Eastern Europe—they are sometimes shocked we have internet."

In the years after the Szilágyis had decamped to Sopron, the range of high-value procedures available to dentists expanded. Since 600 A.D., when the Mayans began replacing their mandibular teeth with shell shards, human beings have been inserting materials into their jaws in the hopes that bone would grow around them and fix the foreign object in place. (This is different from dentures, like the chimerical wooden teeth history has placed in George Washington's mouth, which merely fill the voids created by lost or removed incisors.) Over the years, the substances changed, depending on what was available, the ease with which they adhered to the jawbone, and what was durable enough to survive daily use. According to Baylor University periodontist Celeste M. Abraham, author of an admiring history of the procedure, the materials used ranged from gold ligature wire, shells, ivory, chromium, and cobalt, to iridium and platinum. In the 1960s, surgeons began experimenting with space-age chemical compounds and obscure metallic alloys that could be molded to function as a screw. Such factory-made implants proved easy to decontaminate and sterilize, but their smooth surfaces lacked the grooves and ridges along which bone-forming cells can adhere. Manufacturers had to use acids to etch patterns in those surfaces to facilitate the process that doctors call osseointegration.

Inserting these implants into the jaw was a task beyond the conventional dentist, and required the expertise of a dedicated specialist in oral surgery. A surgeon often had to begin by strengthening the jaw, grafting onto it new bone taken from elsewhere on the patient's body and transplanted into the mouth. Once the surgeon determined there was an expanse of jawbone at once thick and soft enough to pocket an implant, he or she cut through the covering of gums and screwed the metal post of the implant into it. The site was given time to heal, and the implant to integrate into the jaw. Then the surgeon placed atop it a support platform known as an abutment that received

46   the crown, a prosthetic tooth intended to be the only part of the contraption outwardly visible.

Innovations in the field of maxillofacial (a showy term for jaw and face) surgery have not only increased the success rate for implants—measured by whether the jaw accepts the titanium ingot and grows around it the way it would natural bone—but created a range of specialized services and products at different price points. Crowns that more closely resembled human teeth became luxury goods, over which dentists could haggle over exclusive contracts with manufacturers that could be used as a trophy before high-end consumers.

While technology had reduced the healing time necessary after the new tooth had been successfully inserted in the jaw, an implant procedure still typically required at least three visits per patient. There was a preparatory session, often including extraction of decayed teeth; the treatment itself; and a post-surgical examination and subsequent monitoring to confirm that the bone and tissue were growing properly around the artificial tooth. "If you need an implant you need to be committed, because it's a process," says Krisztina Komjáthy, an expert in pharmacoeconomics who serves as managing director of the consultancy Pearl Hungary.

Unlike orthodontic care, which requires patients to return for monthly follow-up visits, a monomaniacal focus on implantology lends itself to economies of scale. It also emboldened egos more commonly identified with heart surgeons than the neighborhood dentist. "It's the same dentistry, but not the same—because you need to focus on the big work," says Attila Kaman, whose Implant Center grew to encompass sixty employees. It was slowly taking over an Art Deco apartment building in a posh quarter of Buda where Kaman chose to decorate his office and conference room with trophies from his hunting trips, including ibex horns from Kyrgyzstan and a taxidermied polar bear from Canada. "The average experienced dentist or surgeon in the UK does in one year 100 implants. I do 2,000 implants," says Kaman.

In 2006, with the goal of reducing the number of international trips patients would have to make as part of their treatment plan, Kaman opened an office in London to offer after-care services to patients who had had surgery at his Implant Center. Not long thereafter, Bátorfi developed his own London presence and traveled there monthly to perform a day's worth of consultations each month in an office he rented from another Hungarian dentist. While Bátorfi offered free diagnostic appointments in Budapest, he charged 45 pounds for the same consultations in London, a fee that was refunded if patients arranged to commence treatment within two months. "It's unknown in the west—the free treatment," he marvels.

As early as 2007, officials within Hungary's Ministry for National Economy had begun thinking about a role for the government in corralling the sector's promising growth. "We feel they do not have enough knowledge about business things. Medical universities do not teach dentists business," says Anikó Kabai, senior lawyer at the Managing Authority of Operational Programme for Economic Development. A survey conducted by Kabai's department counted approximately 6,000 dentists in Hungary, about 10 percent of them committed to the tourist market. "The usual way was that there was only a dentist and he didn't have a manager," Kabai says. "They

48   were a one-man show, but there was not an organized, common framework for them."

Hungary's governments had developed other clusters
around the production of wine, software development, and
wooden furniture. In each instance, officials saw an opportunity to organize firms vertically based on shared strategic interest and interdependence, even if their business models were so
disparate that no common tax or regulatory policy could affect
them all. (The wine cluster might include vineyards and label
printers and companies that clean up pesticide run-off.) More
importantly, the clusters represented an effort to marshal the
energy within the country's most promising economic sectors so that it was directed outward toward foreign competitors
rather than against local rivals. As such, a cluster policy offered
a way for Hungary's government to shift the most important
unit of economic activity from the firm to the nation. "We need
to put together a domestic supply and an international demand,"
says Ádám Ruszinkó, the economic ministry's deputy state sec-
retary for tourism. "In Hungary, the willingness of cooperation
is very low. The Hungarian professions need to learn each other's thoughts to create a common path."

When the Fidesz party returned to government after
the 2010 elections, that became a matter of national priority.
"Dental tourism will play a major role in overcoming public debt
of the last eight years," László Szűcs told the publication *Blikk*
in the spring of 2011. After the new prime minister asked his
dentist to make a presentation to the economic ministry about
how such a program of cooperation might be organized, Bátorfi
dispatched Szűcs on a research mission.

Szűcs found clinics happy to talk, and nearly 600 of them did. Hungary's dentists may have been wary of entrusting their secrets with Bátorfi but they did recognize that his relationship with the prime minister had positioned him to redefine medical tourism in accordance with his ambitions. "The incident caused outrage in the sector overall," *Heti Világgazdaság* reported after Orbán and Szűcs signed the cooperative pact in 2011 before a crowd of 200 dentists. "It's difficult for the profession overall to understand that while the government makes hundreds of millions of forints in budget cuts to the health sector, and rejects the rhetoric of the presence of private capital in the sector, why just one private service was awarded a billion-forint gift."

Some of the money went directly to Bátorfi's Medical Tourism Office, and its subsidiary Hungarian Dental Tourism Development Office, which developed promotional materials and offered training and joint-marketing initiatives. The Medical Tourism Office developed a common website, with a directory of Hungarian dentists looking to promote themselves abroad, and a phone line to handle inquiries and counsel possible customers. "As I see our mission, it's to get people to understand this is not just a price negotiation. It's much more than that," says Zsolt Lakatos, the CEO of Photel, a Budapest-based customer-service contractor that manages the dental program's call center, where as part of their training, operators read British media coverage of dental tourism as a lens onto the often conflicted views prospective patients have about traveling to Hungary. "Our job is to make sure we convince you that for that operation you need to come here."

50   The rest of the money, through a government grant scheme using European Union funds, went to individual dentistries. Approximately three hundred of them, the majority in Budapest, qualified to apply—apparently by paying membership dues to the Medical Tourism Office. (The monthly dues were 180,000 forints, or about 670 dollars, with a discounted annual rate.) Along with Estonia and the Czech Republic, Hungary receives the most subsidies per capita from the European Union, a transfer of wealth that some have likened to the Marshall Plan. Restrictions on use of the funds—they couldn't pay for real estate or wages, commonly the most significant expenses a clinic faces—grated dentists, but few had a choice. Thirty-nine dentists ended up winning grants in 2012, for between 16 and 30 million forints each, usually to pay for new equipment. In at least one case, a dentist used the grant to purchase plasma TVs for his office, on which he showed Medical Tourism Office marketing videos.

In a sense, Bátorfi was trying to use the government stimulus as a lure to restructure the economics of his field, which had been shaped by the unhealthily merged traditions of Hungarian medicine and the culture of the commission-driven tourist industry. The Medical Tourism Office had designed itself to replace the economic actors known in Hungary as "hawk patient intermediaries." Those agents—like the contact who had sent Bátorfi his first British patients in 2000—could claim one-third of all revenue as a finder's fee. Bátorfi's Medical Tourism Office would fulfill many of the same functions and charge dentists only 15 percent for each referral, gradually decreasing the commission to 10.5 percent by 2017. By setting up new computerized billing systems to produce uniform invoices, the Medical Tourism Office hoped to win the trust of foreign insurers who had been wary of sending their patients abroad to receive treatment plans that they couldn't quite decipher. Along the way, Bátorfi would fix what might be the biggest challenge to his profession's economic growth, which was that, by his own estimate, "Fifty percent of this field is on the black market."

Brain Drain

In 2006, the administrators of Kútvölgyi Hospital, the teaching institution of Semmelweis University, the oldest medical school in Hungary, summoned one of their faculty members and asked if he could help make them money. Throughout the period of Soviet domination, the Bauhaus-style structure perched on a ridge high above Buda had been the place top officials of Hungary's communist party and government had gone for their medical care. Like many of the country's public hospitals, Kútvölgyi had struggled after the fall of the Berlin Wall as Hungary adjusted to offering socialized medicine in a free-market economy.

Medical tourism among dental clinics like Béla Bátorfi's thrived in that environment. Hospital officials began to look upon the nascent sector with some disdain. After all, doctors who performed the least essential services were the most likely to thrive within it, while public hospitals were forced to contend with tight budgets in a highly regulated market. Resentment turned to envy, then eventually to practical curiosity. Kútvölgyi executives summoned Gábor Szócska and wanted answers to one question: Was medical tourism any more than a fad?

Szócska was an internist by training but devoted his career to what amounted to a form of health-care trend-spotting. He was in medical school as Hungary emerged from Soviet domination, earning his diploma in 1990. As Hungary changed economic systems he took an interest in the way that the country's health-care administration would adjust along with it. After a postgraduate degree in medical management from the London School of Hygiene and Tropical Medicine, Szócska sought a degree in medical management at Semmelweis. He returned to Budapest with the intent to study how fledgling hospitals were faring after being spun off from the state-owned system.

By 2006, the medical-tourism sector was ready for similar examination. It did not take long for Szócska to discover that the most commonly accepted claims about the exceptional scope of Hungarian dentistry were baseless. The mythology had been created by a British press entranced by superlatives, and the new celebrity-dentists they had crowned in Budapest found little reason to challenge it. Even with the massive growth in the professional ranks since 2008, Hungary didn't have that many dentists—only one for every 2,000 citizens. That figure placed it below the European Union average of 1.32, and amounted to half as many as the continent's leader, Iceland. Hungary's per-capita ratio, in line with Switzerland's and Slovakia's, appeared "satisfying" to domestic needs, Szócska concluded, but didn't

54   indicate that Hungary's market position derived simply from a surfeit of supply.

Following the money was more difficult. While plenty of revenue from dental tourism seemed to be flowing effortlessly into Hungary, no one seemed to know how much of it there was, where exactly it was coming from, or where it was ending up. The very nature of a practice that fell between, or across, national regulatory régimes made it hard to confidently track or measure, and significantly cramped both academic and industry research on the subject worldwide. As most of the foreign dental patients coming to Hungary were paying out-of-pocket, governments and insurers in their home countries were unable to track their spending.

Szócska enlisted a younger colleague at Semmelweis, Eszter Kovács, who had studied health sciences with a research interest in the mobility of health professionals within Europe. When the two polled Hungary's dentists (or at least the 273 who responded to a survey) they found that despite the overseas visibility of the clinics catering to tourists, their activity represented only a niche activity within Hungarian dentistry. Only 24 percent of the dentists reported serving any foreigners within their patient base. From within that group only half of those said that in an average month, they treated primarily foreigners. "Why is Hungary the main destination country in dental tourism?" Szócska and Kovács asked, in what became the title of a paper they co-authored with two other colleagues. "Why do patients choose Hungary for dental care?"

Hungary was indisputably inexpensive, its costs for treatment in line with Mexico's, generally above Costa Rica's and below Thailand's. When compared across countries, fees appeared to be far more stable for crowns—where a significant share of the cost is associated with the relatively fixed price of the raw materials—than a service like whitening, which was more dependent on labor costs and could be five times more expensive in the United Kingdom than in Thailand or India. (Fees in the United States were almost exactly midway between the two.)

Overwhelming majorities of patients were coming on private journeys as opposed to organized trips, relying more than anything else on word of mouth to shape their decisions. Price was the filter that led foreigners to Hungary, Szócska concluded, while personal recommendations directed them to choose individual dentists. "Friends' recommendation is the most trustworthy source; good experiences generate more and more satisfied patients," Szócska and Kovács wrote. Dentists believed that the biggest problem with serving tourists, Szócska and Kovács learned, was that distance made it difficult to monitor and follow up with patients the way they would with locals. "Time pressure leads us to overtreatment and aftercare," they concluded.

Armed with this understanding of the business's strengths and weaknesses, Szócska persuaded Kútvölgyi administrators to grant him use of an abandoned section of the building to test his theories in the marketplace. He developed a new brand, Kútvölogyi Premium, that would distinguish the foreigner-centric private practice he was building from the rest of the hospital's business. He recruited Tamás Korchmáros,

56   a Hungarian dentist who had worked for ten years in Vienna, and his wife Réka, a periodontist, and outfitted a state-of-the-art clinic for them. Semmelweis already had a dental practice, but it had developed a deficit of 100 million forints and a set of books that were impossible to penetrate. "After that we had to start something new that will solve this problem," says Tamás Korchmáros.

At first, a lot of that was marketing, which was outside the typical tool kit of Hungarian medical administrators. Szócska created a stand-alone company, Premium Healthcare International Hungary, that could partner with other tourism businesses to develop promotional packages to expand Kútvölgyi's customer base. For 195 euros, a would-be patient would get a round-trip ticket from any one of seventeen cities in northern or western Europe and a one-night hotel stay to visit what online display ads for the promotion called the "City of Teeth." (When Kútvölogyi offered a three-day package that included airfare and three-star accommodations, Szócska says he found "tourists coming to Budapest with absolutely perfect teeth because it was a good price for three days in Budapest.")

Those who followed through on the examination and received the free "mouth-hygiene management plan" included in the deal found a small clinic trying to bridge the appeal of a boutique practice with the benefits of a large institution. Kútvölogyi Premium Dental had its own entrance so patients did not have to confront the sights and smells of a working hospital as they entered and exited, but while in the dental chair they had the peace of mind knowing that the phone line in the operating room connected immediately to resuscitation

services. "We are a real dental clinic," says Tamás Korchmáros.
"Not in a hotel."

Under Szócska's guidance, the Korchmároses experimented with many of the techniques other dental-tourism outfits used to bring clients to Budapest. They maintain a patient room in Bristol, where a Hungarian-born dentist performs consultations on their behalf, and have relied on agents, although they limit their commission to twenty percent. ("I know agents who get more money than the dentist," Tamás scoffs.)

Generally, however, Kútvölogyi Premium Dental has eschewed some of the flashier forms of self-promotion. "We don't believe in marketing. It is a very good business for the marketing man, but not for me," he says. "The only good marketing for me is a patient of mine tells two or three or five other people."

The most dramatic business decision they've made has been to resist any desire to mimic the Bátorfi or Kaman model of dental tourism. From the beginning, the Korchmároses insisted on serving local patients, fully aware that, as Tamás acknowledges, "only the implants will result in a high income, not the smaller treatments." (Even so, because agents take commissions out of many foreign patients' fees, they do not always deliver higher levels of income than domestic ones.) Although laws require clinics to charge foreign patients the same as Hungarian citizens, Korchmáros is permitted to establish mutual agreements—hospital employees and their families get a 50-percent discount, for example—that serve to keep prices down for non-tourists. "We have lots of business agreements

with all patients separately," he says with a wink. "We are trying to keep this method in the legal area." Today over half of his
patients are Hungarian. He thinks it may be a signal of quality to his foreign clientele—"when we are traveling in Italy
we are looking for the places crowded with Italian citizens"—
but more importantly the diverse portfolio serves as a hedge
against the vicissitudes of the global marketplace.

Szócska grew convinced that they had arrived at a potential
free-market solution to their greatest long-term concern: the
stability of the country's health-care sector. "Dental tourism is
mutually beneficial to the international patients and the institutions, namely increases investments and stimulates doctors," Szócska and Kovács concluded in one paper.

Encouraged by the success of the dental practice, Szócska
considered expanding the range of specialties offered under the
Kútvölgyi Premium banner. The dynamics of dentistry were
distinct from other aspects of medicine: the industry had been
private for a decade already, breeding an entrepreneurial culture among dentists and an understanding of how to market
themselves in a competitive marketplace. It might take more
work to prepare other doctors for the experience of dealing
with medical tourists, but the same dynamics that brought
dental patients to Budapest could apply to other parts of a hospital. The hospital agreed to hand over seven patient rooms for
use by medical tourists, and Szócska imagined renovating the
entire model of the Hungarian hospital.

St. John's Hospital is one of the most prestigious institutions
to endure from fin-de-siècle Budapest, but the sole part of it

that the city's healthy residents usually see is the handsome redbrick façade belonging to the main administration offices, facing a thoroughfare in Buda's District XII. When the building opened in 1898, St. John's had only five departments, including those covering pediatrics and basic surgery. Over the next few decades, the St. John's campus grew to incorporate other specialized practices—eye care, orthopedics, venereal-urology—and the new structures to house them, along with an X-ray laboratory. (It is known in Magyar as Szent Janos.) World War II constrained its ambitions, although the hospital was not directly attacked. After the war, Hungary's medical facilities were nationalized by the country's new Soviet-controlled government. Under the communist system, health care became an entitlement, with nearly every Hungarian citizen receiving free coverage from government hospitals staffed by public employees. As a result, the total number of per-capita hospital beds in Hungary nearly doubled between 1938 and 1965.

That expansion of coverage may have come at the cost of Hungary's relative medical sophistication. "Most of the hospital facilities are old and often obsolete," as Yale medical school and hospital administrator Edwin Richard Weinerman concluded after an Eastern European study tour under the auspices of the World Health Organization in April 1967. "They are equipped with the essentials of modern scientific care but with few of the semi-luxuries that add to quality and convenience," Weinerman observed of Hungarian hospitals at a variety of sizes and levels. "Patient accommodations are crowded, generally unaesthetic, and lacking in provision for personal privacy, although they are clean and well supervised and have a warm

60   and friendly atmosphere as far as relations between patients
and nurses are concerned."

Today the assessment is even more dismal, Szócska
explains while descending the ridge from his office one floor
below the Kútvölgyi Premium Dental Clinic toward the tram
interchange of Széll Kálmán Square. As he walks through
the warren of buildings on the St. John's campus it is easy to
imagine that little has changed since Weinerman's visit. But
unlike Weinerman, who accompanied doctors on their rounds
to assess the quality of the Hungarian health system, Szócska
doesn't even need to enter any hospital buildings to illustrate
what's wrong with it. Instead the evidence is in St. John's park-
ing lots. On one stretch of pavement, Szócska gestures pityingly
to the spaces reserved for employees of the pathology department. One is filled by a Hyundai, the other a compact Renault.

In the more posh residential districts of Buda or the livelier
tourist precincts of Pest, private clinics are recognizable from
the street because the cars parked by the dentists, plastic surgeons, and gynecologists who work inside are often Porsches
or BMWs.

Medical tourism has helped to subsidize many of the payments on those sports cars, but the fundamental class divide
among Hungarian medical professionals—between those working in its public hospitals and those in private clinics—has its
origins in the socialized medicine of Hungary's communist era.

Nearly all medicine in Hungary was controlled from Department 6 of the Health Ministry in Budapest. There bureaucrats received budgets and performance reports from public

municipal, county, regional, and national hospitals, which together employed every Hungarian doctor. (Doctors were required to work for the state.) After the data had been processed by Department 6, it was handed off to the National Planning Office, where 500 employees sharing an ICL 4-70 mainframe computer produced the five-year plans that Hungary used to manage its entire economy. It was a system that by most measures proved relatively efficient as it guaranteed health coverage to nearly every citizen. By 1980, Hungary had attained admirably high rates of per-patient visits to doctors (5.4 annually) and average stay for admitted patients (fifteen days) while keeping its national health-care spending impressively low (only 4.6 percent of GDP).

The only medical activity in Hungary beyond the control of Department 6 usually took place in doctors' apartments and houses. Once they had completed their quota of public work, government doctors were free to spend one hour per day serving private patients. (Salaries, paid by the state, were determined by a doctor's experience, academic degrees, and the characteristics of the geographic district in which he or she practiced.) Because full-scale private enterprise was restricted, doctors had to serve patients from their homes. Treatments there were subject to regulated rates, although doctors were subsidized through a practice Hungarians call *hálapénz*, meaning "money in envelopes," a payment somewhere between a tip and a bribe for better or faster attention. At one point, 4,000 out of Hungary's 25,000 doctors maintained some sort of private practice.

In 1989, Hungary rewrote its constitution to ensure that, amid the transition to capitalism, "people living within the

62   territory of the Republic of Hungary have the right to the high-
      est possible level of physical and mental health." Freely elected
      leaders disbanded the National Planning Office, but maintained
      a system of socialized medicine for citizens, who would make
      an annual payroll tax contribution to subsidize it. Instead of
      setting doctors' salaries, the health ministry would regulate the
      medical sector through a fee-for-service model in which
      the government would maintain a list of approved procedures.
      When a hospital performs one of the procedures, it applies
      for reimbursement from a national compulsory insurance
      pool, which typically covers the entire expense of the treat-
      ment. A Hungarian citizen can count on her government to
      pay for a life's worth of necessary medical care, often without
      demanding a co-pay for anything other than some medications
      and prosthetics.

      Yet to manage the cost to taxpayers of such a generous sys-
      tem, the government caps the number of procedures for which it
      will pay each hospital annually. This "volume control" succeeded
      in controlling the pay of doctors and nurses. With a hospital's
      revenue limited by the number of reimbursed procedures it could
      perform, Hungarian doctors never saw their salaries rise the way
      that members of other professional classes did. In 2006, the aver-
      age salary for health-industry employees was barely 75 percent of
      the sector-wide average for Hungarian white-collar workers.

      That meant that doctors who maintained private practices
      thrived more than ever. There is a "strong tradition of under-
      the-table money," or *hálapénz*, Szócska says. "Gynecologists are
      rich doctors now, but unofficially. The dentists are rich, too," he
      observes. "Plastic surgeons are going the same way as dentists."

The same European integration that had accelerated the organic growth of Hungarian dental tourism also posed the greatest challenge to the stability of the country's health-care system. In 2003, the country's voters had decided overwhelmingly to join the European Union, opening Hungary's borders to the continent's growing common markets.

Upon acceding to the EU, many Eastern European countries have had to contend with what policymakers call a "brain drain." Without limits on inter-European migration, talented professionals decamped westward in search of jobs, quality of life, and adventure.

In Hungary, that phenomenon has been felt particularly in the medical sector, because the insurance regulations serve to limit the pay of any doctor working within the public system. It has been a problem since the days of Department 6, when doctors who could replicate their clinics at home were able to make money on the side. Gynecologists, obstetricians, and dentists all found this easy. Those who relied on hospital infrastructure and staff support—like heart surgeons—were left helpless and had no options to claim additional income domestically. "Many of the Hungarian doctors go abroad because salaries are higher in Western Europe," says Kovács. "But dentists stay, because they can have that salary here if they desire."

To illustrate the possibility, Szócska walked farther down Swabian Hill from his office to a converted sanatorium that now houses Semmelweis's Heart and Vascular Center. Only two facilities in Europe perform more heart transplants, and it is the Hungarian government that forestalls Semmelweis from doing more.

Heart disease has long been the chief cause of death for Hungarians, but public money at Semmelweis runs out after about 1,800 pacemaker implants. As a result of those regulations, 20 percent of the cardiology center's beds typically go unoccupied.

The roots of the Hungarian medical brain drain can be traced to those empty beds across the country's hospitals. The lost revenue they represent serves to effectively limit what hospital administrators can budget for doctors' salaries and the training, conference travel, and new equipment that would convince doctors that they could grow in their jobs. "If you're in a country with economic troubles, like Hungary, you have limited budgets," says Béla Merkley, the chair of Semmelweis's Heart and Vascular Center. "It's really important to increase other types of moneys."

For years, facilities like Semmelweis have often done so by administering clinical studies on behalf of medical-device manufacturers or drug trials for pharmaceutical companies, which have seemingly limitless research budgets when pursuing potentially lucrative innovations. (After federal disclosures showed that it had paid $287.4 million to American doctors and teaching hospitals in 2014, Pfizer told *Wall Street Journal* that more than three-quarters of the payments were for costs associated with clinical trials.)

But the dental clinic up the hill introduces Merkeley to a viable method of funding that is more within the hospital's control. Every time he can fill one of those beds with a patient who lacks Hungarian national insurance, Merkeley stands to not only justify the extra capacity but—by generating revenue not constrained by government regulations—funds what in effect amounts to a parallel discretionary budget.

Semmelweis's Heart and Vascular Center has several advantages competing for patients in the marketplace for medical tourists. Its doctors perform coronary catheterizations for about 5,000 euros, less than one-fifth what they would cost in Germany. (The minimally invasive procedure involves inserting a thin tube into the heart.) One reason the costs are so low is the reduced pay earned by Hungarian doctors: Even Merkeley, who has served as Semmelweis's head of cardiology since 2003, earns just 2,000 euros in salary each month. Merkeley is an accomplished specialist and chair of the clinic, rumored to be the next chancellor of his country's most prominent medical school, whose office décor attests to his service as the doctor for several of his country's sporting federations. Given the hours he works there, however, Merkeley makes about as much as a Wal-Mart greeter under the company's newly elevated minimum wage for its American employees.

But Semmelweis is not drawing Germans looking for a bargain the way that Kútvölgyi's dental practice might, nor is it luring wealthy Saudis away from Bavarian hospitals with competitive pricing. Instead, the foreign cardiology patients are from countries to Hungary's south and east—Serbia, Croatia, Macedonia, Romania, and Kazakhstan among them—that lack specialists to serve the cardiovascular needs of the local population. Because, unlike many of the cosmetic procedures that previously defined Eastern European medical tourism, treating an acute heart attack is not considered to be elective, a patient's domestic insurer typically assumes the cost. With patients

66   rarely paying out-of-pocket for, say, a cardiac MRI, according to
      Merkeley, "this is not a question of the price; they pay what we
      ask for."

      He describes medical tourism as effectively a wealth trans-
      fer to subsidize Semmelweis's core mission. "We are a big clinic
      and we concentrate mostly on Hungarian patients. These extra
      activities are mostly for having a little more money and having
      more profile worldwide," says Merkeley. "We finance for the care
      of Hungarians with help from treating foreign people." Merkeley
      says he distributes the increased revenue not only among his cen-
      ter's 135 doctors, but to the nurses and assistants, too. At least in
      his rarified corner of the Hungarian health-care system, medical
      tourism has helped to stanch the brain drain. Since he became the
      cardiovascular center's director in 2011, Merkeley boasts, "only
      one colleague went to the United States and never came back."

      In Merkeley's view, this is a virtuous cycle, in which for-
      eign revenue permits a public hospital like Kútvölgyi to main-
      tain a higher quality and greater range of specialized care than
      could ever be supported by direct or indirect funding from
      domestic sources. The Croatian government has contracted
      with Semmelweis to perform ablation procedures for which
      Zagreb's hospitals are unsuited. This is a familiar arrangement
      to the Hungarian medical sector, although historically the coun-
      try was a buyer of such services rather than a seller of them. The
      country's national insurer currently pays the Austrian govern-
      ment for its hospitals to administer pulmonary transplants to
      Hungarian citizens.

      Beyond such contracts, there has been little direct govern-
      ment intervention to make this possible. Instead, Semmelweis

happens to find itself conveniently positioned at a meeting of
local supply and global demand that fortuitously manages to
not only make business sense but serve a public-policy interest.
"How can we improve the Hungarian medical system to opti-
mize it for health tourism?" asks Szócska. "We need to improve
the possibility of Hungarian medical tourism and we need to
improve the treatment of Hungarian patients, too."

Flying Bodies

In 2010, a reporter for the Israeli newspaper *Haaretz* donned the fictional identity of a sixty-year-old foreign woman and called the Sheba Medical Center—the Middle East's largest hospital, located near Tel Aviv—to inquire about having a growth on her kidney removed. Israel's state comptroller had recently issued a report on waiting times for hospital appointments, and determined that it would take two or three months for a sixty-year-old Israeli woman to schedule an appointment for diagnostic work and treatment at Sheba. (The wait for an ear, nose, and throat operation at Nahariya's Medical Center of the Galilee, the government researchers concluded, was thirteen months.)

By some measures, Israel has an immensely successful health system: average life expectancy is 81.7 years and the country spends only 7 percent of its GDP on health. Based largely on these figures, Bloomberg in 2014 ranked Israel's as the world's seventh most efficient national health-care system;

the United States, by contrast was 44th out of 51 developed
countries surveyed. (American life expectancy is 78.7 years, at
the cost of over 17 percent of GDP.)

But to reach such efficiency the Israeli patient experience
suffered dramatically: The country's four-day average hospital
stay was well below average among nations in the Organisation
for Economic Co-operation Development, as was its ratio of
only two hospital beds per thousand residents. "Among OECD
nations," noted *Haaretz*, "only Mexico fares worse."

Prompted by the comptroller's report, the newspaper
launched its own investigation to pinpoint some blame for
hospital overcrowding. At the time Israel received an estimated 30,000 medical tourists, many coming from the former
Soviet Union because of the low costs of Israeli care. Others
from neighboring countries traveled to Israel for specific procedures they couldn't get from skilled specialists at home; every
patient in Cyprus who requires a bone-marrow transplant has
to leave the island. In 1995, the Health Ministry issued a directive declaring that such tourism could not come at the expense
of Israeli patients, although that diktat (which included no
new rules for hospitals) did not slow the enthusiasm among
both public and private sector officials to market Israel as
a destination for foreign patients. "Advocates of medical tourism," *Haaretz* acidly observed, "include virtually the entire
medical establishment."

Haaretz learned that hospitals were doing more to bring in
patients they called "flying bodies" than merely advocating for
the practice. Public hospitals contracted with so-called health
corporations to manage their business with private customers,

including foreigners. There were "separate lines" for tourists, a hospital operator confided in the newspaper's fictional sixty-year-old foreign woman, with several time slots per day earmarked for them. "You tell me a week before you're arriving and I'll arrange everything," Sheba's representative told the undercover journalist. "Generally, the operation takes place within a few days."

In November 2010, the newspaper concluded its investigation and reported that "medical tourists to Israel enjoy medical conditions Israelis can only dream of." In so doing, *Haaretz* managed to juxtapose the failure of the government—then led by Benjamin Netanyahu's center-right party—to efficiently deliver promised social services to its own citizens, with its promotion of medical tourism as part of an economic-growth strategy. Even though *Haaretz* could not demonstrate a causal connection, the suggestion that the two dominant trends in the country's health-care economy might be linked amounted to an indictment that the medical establishment was chasing profits at the expense of people it was supposed to serve.

In countries with less-developed medical sectors than Israel's, medical tourism could be blamed for even more catastrophic damage. When West African medicine became the focus of international attention during the 2014 Ebola outbreak there, many saw medical tourism—and the fact that local elites chose to opt out of domestic hospitals by heading abroad—as a culprit for the underfunded condition of the region's public-health infrastructure. Al-Jazeera noted that Nigerians spent nearly $500 million annually to pay for care abroad, primarily in India, Egypt, the United Kingdom, and the United Arab

Emirates. "There are people that have sold their houses in order to take somebody to India for treatment," Mike Egboh, the national program manager for the Partnership for Transforming Health Systems, told the network. That exodus could trigger a vicious cycle: the existing hospital system was being starved of revenues, and Nigeria's most promising doctors were forced to seek jobs overseas, primarily in the United States, leaving domestic hospitals without a local constituency for investment and reform.

As it has since independence, Nigeria's government extends free and subsidized medical care to citizens, but does not have the type of health services to sustain that promise. According to University of Lagos College of Medicine neurology professor Mustapha Danesi, more than 90 percent of Nigerians go to government hospitals, but only 10 percent of doctors are paid by those facilities. Those who choose to go to foreign ones are certainly not doing so in search of bargains; the other choices for them would be to join the long lines of Nigerians waiting for attention from hospitals unable to serve them, or to pay out of pocket at a private hospital. Instead, they are traveling as a rational response to a health-care system that is, in Danesi's words, "under-developed rather than decadent."

To make medical tourism a target for those who criticize the state of domestic health care, one has to consider it a finite resource rather than one whose scarcity is determined by political decisions. Israel, a relatively prosperous country that has quickly made itself a global leader in biotech innovation, has explicitly chosen to make cost control a priority over patient convenience.

After *Haaretz*'s report, others were encouraged to probe the excesses of medical tourism in Israel. An undercover team from Channel 2 filmed three surgeons at Tel Aviv's Ichilov Hospital soliciting under-the-table payments from a travel agency promoting medical tourism, ostensibly to prioritize operations on foreign patients. A Finance Ministry audit revealed doctors billing to perform procedures on medical tourists as they simultaneously collected salaries for their work on the government payroll, relying on hospital facilities like imaging centers and laboratories to complete the private work on public time. Other Ichilov doctors told Channel 2 they had seen patients given unnecessary procedures purely because of the revenue it generated for their hospitals. Some of these investigations found medical professionals involved in clearly unethical behavior, in certain cases likely also illegal. (The three Ichilov surgeons were suspended by their hospital the day after Channel 2 aired its footage, and the Tax Authority subsequently investigated them for crimes including employee theft and bribery.) In most instances, however, doctors and hospital administrators were responding rationally to the peculiar incentives that Israel's health-care system imposes on them. At 3:00 p.m., doctors leave the government payroll, and can choose either to go to the beach or to tend to private patients. Treating an Israeli with public funds at that time of day is not an option.

But the government's response to the growing medical-tourism scandal did not address the underlying cause, which would have almost certainly required—whether through taxes, fees, or co-pay—making Israeli citizens pay more for expanded services. Instead, one week after the Channel 2 report, the

Health Ministry issued a directive that public hospitals and the health corporations that managed their private business would have to charge foreign and Israeli patients under the same fee schedule, and would be required to pay doctors at the same rate regardless of the patient's nationality. "Medical tourism has grown significantly in recent years, and I see this growth as something problematic, also being pushed by business interests," explained the ministry's director general, Ronni Gamzu, as he unveiled the new rules before a Knesset committee.

Medical tourism "will be seriously harmed and perhaps even collapse," Rabin Medical Center director Eran Halperin wrote to the ministry. As Halperin noted elsewhere in his letter, effectively cutting off a lucrative source of income to the doctors and technicians who worked there would only motivate them to establish their own private clinics and cater those practices even more narrowly to serve foreign patients. If the health ministry decided to increase co-pays for public hospitals to make up for the lost revenue and discourage overcrowding through higher costs, Israelis might soon find it more cost-effective to travel to Turkey and avoid the waits.

In every case, medical tourism would not be creating new inequities as much as magnifying existing ones. No government policy had the power to cause a collapse in medical tourism, because medical tourism was a fluid concept that adjusted as a response to government policies. Israel's health ministry could certainly set regulations that had the consequence of redirecting traffic—transforming Israel from a destination for medical tourists to a source of them—but no one could anticipate how hospitals and government in Jordan or Cyprus or Tunisia

74   would respond. The challenge of balancing interests across bor-
       ders would fall to something beyond the nation-state, and there
       was only one transnational government on Earth with the legal
       authority and political ambition to try.

Europa

In 1996, Manfred Molenaar and Barbara Fath-Molenaar returned from their home in France to Karlsruhe to sue their insurance company. On January 1, 1995, the couple had begun paying heath-policy premiums to Allgemeine Ortskrankenkasse Baden-Württemberg, in compliance with German law that required individuals to acquire coverage. Mrs. Molenaar was a German citizen, while her husband was Dutch. The two later moved to France. But when they attempted to collect benefits, their insurer told them that they were ineligible to do so because they were no longer German residents. In October 1997, the Molenaars went before the European judges charged with balancing national laws with the continent's principles, to argue that where they lived should have no bearing on the benefits to which they were entitled.

The following year, Germany informed one of its citizens, Friedrich Jauch, that he would no longer receive social-security

76   benefits despite the fact that he had been born in the lake-
      side Bavarian town of Lindau and lived there through all of his
      seventy-one years. For nearly five decades, he had worked just
      across the border in Austria, regularly making contributions to
      an insurance fund, and the German government directed Jauch
      to seek benefits there. But when he turned to Austria's Pension
      Insurance Institution to collect—he had made 480 monthly
      contributions over his lifetime—it ruled he was also ineligi-
      ble for Austrian social-security benefits because he had never
      been an Austrian resident. In 1998, Jauch sued both countries'
      institutions over the limbo in which he found himself: He had
      lived his life straddling a national border and was now, in old
      age, being told that from the vantage of the welfare state he was
      a man without a country.

      The European Court of Justice ruled on behalf of both Jauch
      and the Molenaars, determining that such enforcement of insur-
      ance regulations unreasonably violated their rights to move
      freely within Europe. Starting with the Treaty of Rome, which
      established the European Economic Community in 1958, the
      engineers of continental integration asserted that the formation
      of a common market required respect "four freedoms"—the free
      movement of persons, services, goods, and capital. (While West
      Germany was one of the founding members of the European
      Community, Austria did not join until 1995, when it had been
      transformed into the European Union.) In 2001, the court further
      ruled in favor of a Belgian couple who challenged Luxembourg's
      National Family Benefits Fund, for denial of maternity and child-
      birth allowances because they did not have Luxembourgian resi-
      dency. Basic health benefits to which citizens are entitled, the

court determined over the course of its three opinions, could not
be made contingent on geography.

Together the cases marked a new way of thinking about the
place of health care in Europe. From 1958 onward, governments
had carved out medicine as beyond the reach of their integration.
"Union action shall respect the responsibilities of the Member
States for the definition of their health policy and for the organization and delivery of health services and medical care," reads
the Treaty for the Functioning of the European Union. "The
responsibilities of the Member States shall include the management of health services and medical care and the allocation
of the resources assigned to them." But as the court recognized,
the further integration of member countries' economies made
it harder to reconcile that specific exemption with the promise of a common internal market. "The *Molenaar* and *Jauch* cases
thus exemplify the attempts of Germany and Austria to exempt
their welfare benefits from exportability, and so to speak to con-
struct 'safe havens' in both national and EU law," University of
Copenhagen political scientist Dorte Sindbjerg Martinsen has
written. "Such 'safe havens' may not prove to be lasting firewalls
around national social services in the long run."

When Rostislava Dimitrova arrived in Brussels in 2006, it was
clear how much the European Union's health-care priorities
had changed as a result of those judicial decisions. Dimitrova
was a doctor, but beyond one year in medical school she had
never practiced medicine. Instead, she worked in health policy
in her native Bulgaria, for its health ministry and parliament. In
2005, the country decided to join the European Union, planning

its official entry two years later. Dimitrova was among the bureaucrats dispatched from Sofia initially to serve as a staffer in the European parliament, working on its health committee, before being transferred to a job at the European Commission's Directorate-General for Health and Consumers.

At DG SANCO, as the department was known in Brussels, the cautious undertaking of stitching together Europe's disparate health systems was already underway. In response to the court decisions, the European Commission in 2004 passed a resolution to begin the process. Its result, unveiled two years later, was the European Health Insurance Card, a wallet-sized ID technically issued by one's national insurer for recognition in other European jurisdictions. The card had limited utility, only to facilitate "medically necessary, state-provided health care during a temporary stay," as the EU website says. (The card now also exists as a smartphone app.)

Dimitrova was assigned to work on an EU Health Strategy, which would move from the mostly symbolic creation of an identification card to a deeper integration. Among the recommendations the European Commission adopted for its fledgling E-Health Network was setting standards for health records so that patient files and prescriptions could be transferred and read across borders.

European regulators, however, decided to apply a different set of rules to medical policy than they did to other areas of economic integration, where typically Brussels developed a Europe-wide structure and compelled member states to participate. When it came to health records, the European Union guided the establishment of a voluntary network, where

European bureaucrats offered support but had no real control.
"It would be an empty network if member states did not decide
to join it," says Dimitrova. "It was a very sensitive topic for
member states—they didn't want to give authority to the commission to handle e-health."

National politicians were already conditioned to chafe at
the European Union for creating new continent-wide standards
in areas that had traditionally been subject to local regulations:
consumer protection, agriculture, environmental conserva-
tion. The politics of health care functioned differently, as medical services were treated as a scarce resource nurtured by local
economies, where inevitably foreign winners would produce
local losers. Trying to synthesize a matter as seemingly uncom-
plicated as a tech standard highlighted and intensified existing
inequities among countries.

The politics of the E-Health Network quickly split Europe's
rich countries from its poorer ones. Many Western countries
had invested in proprietary systems developed by their own
vendors and contractors in accordance with national standards,
and were loathe to abandon them or effectively have to start
over. Yet for developing countries in Eastern Europe that had
never digitized health records, the promise of EU funds paying the expense of quickly reaching an international standard
proved immensely appealing.

The E-Health Network and the European Health Insurance
Card, however, were not designed to help medical tourists. Both
of these initiatives were a response to the series of oddball situ-
ations that had presented themselves before judges: the man
with a daily international commute, or the bi-national couple

80   resident in a third state. Workers or tourists who in the course
        of their regular travels ended up having to visit a foreign hospi-
        tal would obviously be served. But at that time, medical tourism
        did not amount to a major economic concern. Only 1 percent
        of Europe's public health spending, a commission study esti-
        mated, went to the practice. (Many of the treatments for which
        patients have been traditionally most likely to travel, such as
        cosmetic procedures, are typically financed by private money.)
        But the existence of medical tourism was still a challenge to the
        philosophical and legal promises of a cosmopolitan continent.
        The European Union permitted, even encouraged, citizens to
        cross borders for schooling or a weekend holiday or even to buy
        a case of wine. If the common market guaranteed a right to carry
        benefits across borders for those whose mobility was forced by
        work or family reasons, why should it not also empower indi-
        viduals who wanted to travel expressly to take advantage of
        Europe's common medical market?

        In March 2007, the European Parliament resolved that it
        could delay action no longer. "Healthcare is still perceived, espe-
        cially from member states, as a national issue," says Dimitrova.
        But, she adds, "many people say, 'why should the EU pronounce
        itself on an issue like how chickens should live, and where they
        should live—and not on patients and health care?'"

        Over the next two years, she and her team at DG SANCO
        worked the Directive on Cross-Border Healthcare, the legis-
        lation to codify the "freedom for the recipients of healthcare,
        including persons in need of medical treatment, to go to another
        Member State in order to receive it there." But it was impossible
        to synchronize national health-care systems. When it came to

offering medical services, government regulations had created
a different set of economic actors in Austria than in Italy, for
example, who each responded to incentives fundamentally at
odds with one another.

The parliamentary report had handed the bureaucrats a few
basic principles, centered around the standard that Europeans
who traveled for medical care were entitled to the same benefits extended to them in the country of their residence or citi-
zenship and that states could insist on prior authorization for
those requiring hospital stays. Providers, meanwhile, would be
forbidden from setting different prices for foreign and domestic
patients and required to provide itemized receipts for care in a
standardized format that would facilitate transparency and the
reimbursement process.

The DG SANCO bureaucrats would have flexibility to determine under what conditions governments could require prior
authorization and what exemptions would be available to ensure
they did not pose undue hurdles to the freedom of movement.
(The key lever turned out to be the definition of "hospital care,"
which could be relaxed or tightened as regulators saw fit.) If the
standards were too loose, Spanish health minister Trinidad
Jiménez warned the EU's Council of Ministers, his government
was worried that it would lose the ability to ensure quality standards for its citizens if they went abroad, and would incur new
costs—around two billion euros annually—as its public health
system had to contend with an expanded patient base.

Spain threatened to block this move to codify patients' rights
and began rallying other nations to back up its threat. The politics
eventually played out in much the same way that the debate over

82   digital medical records had, effectively pitting Europe's welfare-state haves against its have-nots. While patients from Europe's wealthiest countries stood to receive the greatest short-term gain—they, after all, were likely to have the most generous benefits at home and the greatest means for travel—their governments also feared they had the most to lose. "The challenge was big resistance from member states to make this easier for patients to find their way to go abroad," says Dimitrova. "They wanted to protect their procedures and their systems."

In 2010, just before the Christmas holiday, Spain's ambassador reached a deal to drop its opposition. According to the compromise, member states could insist on prior authorization for highly specialized procedures or those requiring extended hospital stays, although not in a way that presented an obstacle for patients with urgent needs. The process would not necessarily be as streamlined as they would find it at home, though, especially for those in Beveridge systems like Great Britain where cash is never exchanged between a patient and clinic or hospital. Patients would have to pay upfront and seek reimbursement—from either a public health service or a private insurer—after they return from the treatment.

That still could not prevent negotiations over the Directive on the Application of Patients' Rights from becoming a battle over the last trappings of the nation-state. The 28 countries in the European Union today share a common defense, currency, trade policy, diplomatic corps, and a wide variety of regulations to ensure consumer and civil rights. There are suggestions that the European Union could solve its current problems with increased fiscal integration to match its common monetary policy. A single flag flies above them all. For those on both the left and right who found national identity in the strength of their governments or the independence of their culture, a health-care system may find itself increasingly prized as a surviving totem of autarky.

"Care is not a commercial, tradable good; it is a basic need for everyone," said Kartika Liotard, a Dutch socialist, one of the directive's most prominent parliamentary critics, who found herself in unexpected alliance with nativist, anti-European representatives like those from the UK Independence Party. "The new EU directive will mean that insurers drive patients abroad in search of cheaper treatment. But patients—especially if they are seriously ill—just need care in their region, close to their family and a doctor who speaks their language. Health tourism will be a logical consequence of this law, with patients from rich countries able to travel to less expensive countries, where they may be given priority over the local, poorer patients."

"Medical tourism" still evoked the opportunistic pursuit of frivolous cosmetic treatments, a politically unsympathetic combination of vanity and bargain-hunting. "We are not trying to promote medical tourism," insisted French representative Françoise Grossetête, of the center-right Union Pour Un Mouvement Populaire, who served as the directive's rapporteur during parliamentary debate. "I'm quite convinced we are not going to see busloads of citizens going from one member state to another. If the treatment abroad is cheaper than at home, only the cost of the treatment will be reimbursed." Indeed, the new rules and DG SANCO's own research did not anticipate large patient flows.

84   Inequities invited what would be the most damning put-down available: "People were saying it is neoliberal," Dimitrova says. In effect, cross-border health-care represented a traditional conflict of liberal values—in this case a government guarantee of equal rights would not ensure equal opportunity. Quite possibly, it would even magnify existing disparities, both among countries and within them. Because patients would be expected to pay upfront for procedures, nothing about the directive changed the fundamental microeconomic reality of medical tourism: To participate, one needed ready access to (often substantial) amounts of cash. "Many patients who go abroad will be privileged," Dimitrova says. "If there's a queue, they will jump the queue." What passed for justice among the European left, she and her commission colleagues remarked caustically to one another, was "equal misery."

In the end, the legislation's passage was never really in doubt. In 2011, the EU Directive on Cross-Border Healthcare took effect.

Yet member states were slow in implementing its recommendations. After two years, the European Commission warned ten of them that they were failing to meet their obligations under the law. In many cases, they had failed to establish a designated "national contact point" that would coordinate between government and the health sector to advise patients of their rights and provide information on reimbursement.

By then, Dimitrova was tiring of life as a European bureaucrat, not least because her husband refused to move to Belgium so they could live in the same place. As her contract with the commission approached its expiration, Dimitrova began to

consider how she might put her knowledge of the new marketplace—and the laws she helped draft to guide it—on behalf of
her home country.

Bulgarians appeared to gain little immediate benefit by the
new law. Their country was one of more than a dozen countries
that had joined the European Union in the years after 2004,
all in central and eastern Europe. Nearly all were less generous
with health care than the EU's core membership, which meant
that Bulgarians who traveled for care were still likely to have to
assume much of the cost themselves. Bulgaria's health ministry
also failed to make available, via its website and other channels,
information about the new protocols it was required to provide
its citizens to guide them through the process of authorization
and reimbursement. (It was one of the national governments
that received warnings from Brussels for falling behind schedule in the directive's implementation.) As a result, just hundreds of Bulgarians took advantage of their new entitlement to
public benefits for medical care abroad. It was a simple fact, said
Dimitrova, that "patients in countries like ours would benefit a
lot less from the directive."

She had spent years struggling with the international politics around medical tourism, and her legacy in that sphere was a
dubious one. "The member states basically hate this directive,"
says Dimitrova. She started to think about medical tourism in
domestic terms, and decided to see if she could make the member state she knew best learn to love her regulatory handicraft.
"Of course this directive changes the market for health care,"
she says, "and should be seen as an opportunity."

The Bulgarian Method

One of the people most excited about Rostislava Dimitrova's return to her native Sofia was Jeni Adarska, who described herself as a cancer-patient consultant. Fifteen years earlier, Adarska had learned she had cancer. Even though at the time she was working at an insurance company, Adarska found the systems into which she was thrust impossible to manage. "It's not easy to be a patient," she says. "When the patient realizes he has cancer, he is absolutely lost. People can't know what they have to do." Once she returned to health, Adarska decided to assist others in the same situation. "My mother was a nurse, from another century," she says, "so I've seen the best of care for people."

Adarska became an advisor and facilitator for Bulgarians dealing with cancer, and an advocate and gadfly on their behalf. Among the options available to them was to travel, under rules that covered the costs associated with specialized treatment, as long as it was for a service not offered in Bulgaria.

Starting in 2009, Adarska helped patients research options and demonstrate to the National Health Insurance Fund that their planned care met the government's standard for international coverage. (Patients had, in essence, to prove a negative: that Bulgaria lacked the necessary expertise or equipment for their procedure.)

It was not until a few years later, stumbling upon the International Medical Tourism Congress while attending a gathering of cancer researchers in Chicago, that Adarska learned there was a name for what she had thought of as her own provisional practice of strategizing over long-distance treatment. As she surveyed the trade-show floor, where many government agencies from around the world promoted themselves as destinations for medical tourism, Adarska concluded that she needed to think about more than the short-term demands of individual patients. "That's when I realized there should be state policy," she reflects, and "how I started assessing what would be Bulgaria's advantages in medical tourism."

Bulgaria had once been a destination for a certain type of wellness tourism. During the 1980s, the country frequently received Arab visitors, who came to the Black Sea region where the cool air was reputed to have curative properties. In the 1990s, rising wealth in Russia led to many of its citizens buying properties around the Black Sea and even opening Russian schools in the region. But the end of the Cold War also led to a collapse of Bulgaria's close relationships with Arab countries, and with it the patients. (The Black Sea remains a magnet for Israeli tourists, usually seeking a summertime respite, to the

88   point that Hezbollah targeted an Israeli tour bus at the airport in the coastal Bulgarian city of Burgas in a 2012 attack that killed seven, including the suicide bomber.)

Bulgaria had experienced little of the cross-border traffic for non-hospital specialties like dentistry and ophthalmology that had introduced the concept of medical tourism to other Eastern European countries. Co-pays for the treatments covered by the National Health Insurance Fund—an examination, two fillings and an extraction per year—were so low that many Bulgarian dentists chose not to work with the public health system. For those whose practices were among the embassies, hotels, and corporate offices of central Sofia—where the patient base was already likely to consist of some foreign visitors and expatriates—there were encouraging reports of an unexpected boom. In 2004, as Bulgaria completed its final negotiations before signing a treaty to finalize entry into the European Union, fifteen dentists who had begun to feel their way to a business model built around foreign patients established the Bulgarian Association of Medical Tourism. "We weren't on the map of medical tourism at all" at that point, says Ventsislav Stoev, former president of a Bulgarian dentists' association.

That presented Bulgarians a chance to sketch a medical-tourism sector on a blank slate. In Hungary, the European Union's directive cross-border health-care jolted an industry that had developed organically over a generation with barely any constraint from government. By the time policymakers in Budapest or Brussels ever tried to impose any order on the business, it was already webbed by existing interests, loyalties and egos that could not be easily unwound. The new regulations had been drafted by European bureaucrats to serve the interests of continental consistency rather than domestic equity or competitiveness. To a profession that had been built on under-the-table payments and promotional deals mysteriously aggregated into hotel-and-airfare packages, the requirement to offer transparent, consistent pricing was a particularly unwelcome jolt.

In Bulgaria, no one would be bound by precedent or incumbency. The country had officially entered the European Union at the start of 2007 and was still adjusting to the hundreds of millions of new visitors and transplants who were now entitled to freely enter and resettle in the country when the cross-border health-care directive took effect. Everyone potentially touched by medical tourism—including doctors, hospital administrators, government officials, and patient advocates—could try to imagine a medical-tourism sector as a coherent national whole rather than scurrying to rejigger existing businesses.

The regulations Dimitrova had helped to draft introduced a new set of peculiar, transnational incentives, particularly for patients from richer countries who could now claim their benefits and go bargain-hunting in Eastern Europe. In Bulgaria, rehabilitation facilities were poised to benefit more quickly than dental clinics. The various European court decisions that clarified the portability of retirement benefits made Bulgaria particularly appealing to pensioners living in generous Scandinavian countries. Once they hit sixty-five years, Swedes receive an average of about three thousand euros monthly from a national social-security fund. Not only might they find the Black Sea climate more temperate than their own, but their

90   benefits would go much farther. "If a Bulgarian goes to the UK,
      they get reimbursed at the meager amount from the Bulgarian
      National Health Insurance Fund," says Anelia Racheva, admin-
      istrative director of Nadezhda Women's Health Hospital. "If a
      Swede comes here they get the money they'd get in Sweden but
      spend it in a low-cost country like Bulgaria."

      While Bulgarian policymakers eagerly welcomed that
      potential transfer of capital from Europe's wealthy north to
      its struggling southeast, they still had to overcome skepticism
      about the foreigners who came seeking value in the country's
      health-care sector. The European Union's directive introduced
      a politically unpopular tension, in which Bulgarians would be
      forced to battle foreigners for access to scarce resources they
      had already paid for with their taxes. "My first priority is not
      targeted to medical-tourism promotion," says Petar Moscov, an
      anesthesiologist who serves as the country's health minister.
      "Our goal is provide a high level of care for Bulgarian citizens."
      Moscov speaks ominously about "the dark side of medical tour-
      ism," intimating that business interests that promote the prac-
      tice have an incentive to maintain health-care disparities. "Why
      in Bulgaria for so many years we don't have these equipment
      items?" he asks. "Is that in someone's economic interest?"

      Adarska considers Moscov a friend, and Dimitrova is a
      consultant to his ministry. Both set out to persuade him that
      improving Bulgaria's standing as a medical-tourism destina-
      tion could be good for Bulgaria's own health care. Residents
      requiring complex treatment were heading abroad. It was a
      source of shame to those who understood that the country had
      made a commitment to provide care to all of its citizens even

as it was technically ill-prepared to deliver on that promise. "Medical tourism offers so much economic leverage," Adarska says. "Our health-care system is hungry for money, and this medical tourism can put money in for the development of our medical system."

If Bulgaria was failing to live up to its pledge of universal health care, it was not simply a matter of lacking infrastructure or capacity. As a legacy of its years under the Soviet-style system, Bulgaria still has one of Europe's highest ratios of hospital beds to population—a report published under the auspices of the World Health Organization described "an excessive and unnecessary use of beds"—but a below-average length of stay for patients. To find a place in the rehabilitation and long-term care centers that were once a source of natural pride, one has to be referred by physicians or the National Social Security Institute. Domestic budgetary concerns, when paired with the loss of foreign visitors from the Middle East, have left one-third of the country's rehabilitation capacity unused, according to Dimitrova's estimate.

The promise of serving patients throughout southeastern Europe was among the factors that led the Tokushukai Medical Corporation to select Sofia over Moscow and Warsaw as the site of its first overseas facility. Since the 2006 opening of Tokuda Hospital, hospital administrators have focused on developing practice areas—including orthopedics, ophthalmology, cardiac surgery, and oncology—whose planned surgeries they determined would be easiest to market to medical tourists. "They are not urgent and can be delayed until you find the best one. You can plan and check where is best for you," says Iavor Drenski,

92 Tokuda's executive director. Within the orthopedic department, hospital administrators assembled a scoliosis center, aware that it would be one of just a handful in Europe. It now draws patients from across the Slavic region, and has developed a framework contract with the Macedonian government to perform complex surgeries on children living there who suffer from spine problems.

At least at Tokuda, some of the promises that Dimitrova and Adarska made to Moscow about the effect that medical tourism could have are being realized. The hospital's pediatrics center now employs eighteen pediatricians, many with narrow specialties sustained only by demand from foreign patients. "For doctors, everyone wants to be unique—all of them, without exception," says Drenski. "Now there is a very free movement of doctors, nurses, and medical staff in Europe. You can imagine how difficult it is for one very small country to keep our doctors here."

Medical tourism has spurred an entrepreneurial spirit into a sector where "during our dark communist time, they said in a public hospital the patient has three rights: to wait, to shut up, and to pay," jokes Drenski. Within the current system, Bulgaria's public and private facilities compete evenly to be reimbursed by the National Health Insurance Fund for treating Hungarian citizens. Charges are set per clinical episode (rather than for individual services) which means patients learn at the time of their consultation how much a treatment will cost and can choose which hospital, public or private, they want to use.

"If they are international patients they are obviously very attractive to us because we get a higher payment," says Ilian

Grigorov, the managing director of City Clinic. City Clinic opened in 2012, and now has three hospitals and is expanding its original structure to 150 beds. A sense of the marketplace informs most of the decisions within: While the company's shareholders include a leading Bulgarian cardiologist and vascular specialist, the hospital's chief administrator is a veteran of the cable-, telecom-, and financial-services sectors.

Still actively disdainful of the push to draw patients from abroad, Moscov is nonetheless attuned to the idea that tourist movement in an open marketplace is a good proxy for quality. He boasts of recent investments in oncology infrastructure, in many cases supported with European funds, and argues that he has succeeded in making unnecessary the type of travel by cancer patients in which Adarska once specialized. "We've done what's needed to stop the flow of medical tourism outside Bulgaria, at least as far as oncology is concerned," Moscov says.

This belated acknowledgment of the fact that Bulgarian health care now competes in a globalized marketplace may have come at just the right time. The fact that the country's hospital system limped through two decades since the end of communism with little structural reform or economic stimulus has left it oddly well-positioned to benefit from new investment interest. "We don't have to deal with legacy buildings, legacy technology," says Grigorov, describing a medical analogue to the sub-Saharan countries able to quickly adopt cell phones in part because they never had to consider it competitive with land lines. Grigorov invokes "evidence-based medicine," a term first coined in the early 1990s to describe practices that supplant clinical judgment with more empirically

94   sound decision-making. "We can go to a generation of technology that's viable for the next ten years. We're developing for the long-term future," he says. "Some of the countries in Eastern Europe have the chance to leapfrog stages of development."

The Eastern Front

Nadezhda Women's Health Hospital had barely been open for two years—in a potentially dismal building on Sofia's outskirts reclaimed from an insurance company and heroically jazzed up for gynecological uses by a television-set designer—before its leadership began talking about expansion. "If the demand starts to go up and up and up, we'll take additional doctors and we'll have the ability to take additional space," says administrative director Anelia Racheva. "That's the advantage of being a private hospital: we chase economic opportunity."

That opportunity could come almost exclusively from medical tourists, who now constitute about one-tenth of Nadezhda's annual flow of about 3,000 patients. While the hospital maintains a waiting list for domestic patients, there is no such delay for foreigners. "There are spots for foreign patients, because we have the guarantee of cash payments," says Racheva. Bulgaria has a number of assets marketing it abroad as a destination for

96   maternity-related services. Hospital prices are about one-third less than in Western European countries, roughly on par with what one pays in Serbia or Croatia. Furthermore, Bulgarian law requires a three-day hospital stay following a natural birth, and four after a Caesarean delivery, for monitoring of both the mother and child. "It's a legacy from old times, that we were in line with Russian standards," Racheva says.

But perhaps the best thing that Nadezdha has going for it is proximity to both Italy and Turkey, two large countries that for reasons informed by very different religious traditions place significant restrictions on access to in-vitro procedures. (Among other criteria, both countries require couples to be married before undergoing an artificial-fertilization process.) Most of the Italian and Turkish women who have made their way to Sofia thus far have done so of their own initiative, but Nadezdha has begun taking steps to appeal more directly to them. Already the hospital has launched an online question-naire, designed to allow foreign patients to assess their suitabil-ity for IVF without having to seek an in-person consultation, and posted in English. Translators are now working on versions in Turkish and German, the latter with an eye toward the large community of Turkish transplants living in Germany.

The unexpectedly colorful atrium of Nadezdha is one of the few places in Europe where Turkey and its increasing influ-ence on the continent's life are discussed with unadulterated cheer. The country bridging two continents stands as an object of fascination and envy, fear and admiration, and resignation that some form of symbiosis will prove necessary. "We com-pare ourselves to Turkey; they are the main destination," says

Ivo Andreev, the marketing manager of City Clinic in Sofia. "They're a model that we follow."

For European nations that have had an ambivalent attitude about promoting inbound medical tourism, Turkey is a striking counter-example of what happens when a country throws itself fully behind the practice. In November 2014, prime minister Ahmet Davutoğlu included medical tourism in a comprehensive plan to modernize Turkey's economy. By 2018, Davutoğlu vowed, Turkey would more than double the number of medical tourists who visited, to 750,000 annually. Revenue from such tourism would increase over three-fold during that period, to $9.3 billion. As was the case with most promises made from Ankara, Davutoğlu's ambition was backed by a powerful central state. Turkey now has a system of so-called free zones for medical tourism, in which all economic activity related to the practice—including construction, doctors' salaries, and investment revenue—is exempt from taxation.

Government officials also welcome medical tourism as part of its broader tourism-promotion campaigns. Turkey is a frequent and prominent participant in health fairs and trade shows around the world, promoting both individual facilities and the national brand. Flag carrier Turkish Airlines extends a variety of promotions (including extra baggage allowance) to patients traveling for medical care. To outsiders, this is the image of an all-powerful government able to pull public and private levers in the service of improving the experience of foreign patients. "If you call #112 anywhere in Turkey and are speaking English, you will be connected right away to an English operator who will direct you to the closest hospital or dentist. And they direct you there by Google Map!" marvels Ventsislav Stoev, chairman of the Bulgarian health-tourism cluster. "Because of the very good example of Turkish medical tourism, we learned it's very important, especially for a small community like ours, to have the support of the government."

Much of this is beyond even the imagination of those in Bulgaria who consider themselves in competition with Turkey for patients. The health ministry, after all, had failed to develop its EU-mandated website advising its own citizens of their options when it came to traveling for care on schedule. Bulgaria Air serves fewer than one-tenth as many destinations as Turkish Airlines. (Hungary no longer even has a national airline.) "The government doesn't care about marketing," says Andreev. "We can't succeed being only one place in a country where there are doubts about services in general, not just medical services." Other countries unable to keep up with Turkey justify the lack of national advertising campaigns to promote medical tourism. "When it comes to the word 'disease' it spells 'disaster' for the tourist industry," says Miodrag Popović, acting director of the Belgrade Tourist Organization in Serbia. "If you're in good health, you don't want to be in the same swimming pool with people who have serious illnesses. No one is promoting medical services in that respect—everyone stops with toothpaste."

Indeed, even when Bulgaria finds competitive advantage it does not derive from a government strategy to develop medical tourism as much as the inadvertent consequence of a benefit created for its own citizens. One decade ago, there were barely 400 in-vitro cycles completed annually in Bulgaria. The

National Health Insurance Fund refused to pay for the procedure, and so Bulgarians who wanted assisted reproduction—
and were able to finance it privately—often ended up traveling
to Greece, which had a more developed medical infrastructure
around it. In 2005, the insurance fund changed its policy, offering partial reimbursement for in-vitro patients, covering the
medications necessary for treatment but not the procedure
itself. In 2009, the Bulgarian government developed a distinct
fund to subsidize the entire cost. It now subsidizes 5,000 couples annually, each of them entitled to three attempts at fertilization. (Genetic testing is not included in the state-funded
package.) Over the decade since the insurance fund's first
tentative steps to embrace in-vitro fertilization, the number
of in-vitro cycles completed in Bulgaria has increased nearly
thirty-fold, to about 11,000 annually. Nadezdha is the largest
of thirty-one medical centers in Bulgaria licensed to practice
artificial fertilization. (Some of the smaller clinics, among them
two located in community hospitals, are responsible for as few
as a dozen cycles a year.)

Today one-third of the babies delivered at Nadezdha come
from in-vitro procedures, and there is reason to believe that
with higher visibility abroad the hospital could draw even more
patients interested in the service. Italy and Turkey are captive
markets, at least as long as they keep their current reproductive
laws, or until a wealthy European nation embarks on an aggres-
sive state-funded campaign to become a destination for IVF
procedures. "The pattern is that patients are traveling east," says
Jeff Coxon, a digital-media strategist who serves as education
and engagement manager for the Medical Tourism Association

100   Europe. "Western Europe is waking up to it now, because they're losing market share."

Indeed, a practice built on policy arbitrage is naturally fraught with uncertainty, although the boldest efforts to regulate the global medical marketplace have created more opportunities for providers than consumers. The EU Directive on Cross-Border Healthcare has made it easier and cheaper for Europeans to travel for care, but also effectively made them less desirable patients elsewhere on the continent. A hospital in an EU country that fills a bed with an EU citizen has to now adhere to a set of regulations that constrain what it can charge and how it has to bill the customer. A non-EU citizen in that same bed can be charged any fee, is not entitled to any transparency in pricing, and has limited legal recourse after the fact. "So private hospitals are more interested in having private patients from Russia or other countries outside Europe," says Rostislava Dimitrova.

There were good cultural reasons for Bulgaria and Hungary to look east for future growth. Both countries had longstanding connections with Russia, to the extent that each found its health-care system still ghosted by Soviet policy choices. When patients are thinking about uprooting themselves at a moment of vulnerability, cultural comfort matters, Gabor Szócska and Eszter Kovács concluded in an article they wrote in collaboration with two Austrian colleagues assessing the dental relationship between their two countries. "Cross-border dental care between Austria and Hungary is unique as strong cultural-historical ties between the two countries and geographical proximity have led to a specialization of dental services," they wrote. Russian citizens have long traveled to Hungarian thermal spas—rumors speculate that Vladimir Putin's helicopter pilot is a regular on Lake Héviz—and find it easy to navigate Bulgaria, which shares Slavic language and traditions.

There certainly were patients to be recruited from Russia. New riches created a demand for high-end cosmetic dentistry that Moscow and St. Petersburg could not easily meet. Russians would not be traveling for cheaper prices or because of local scarcity; they could be lured with promises of specialists skilled in complex procedures. "There is a difference between English and Russian patients," says Béla Bátorfi. "The Russians are more focused on quality." Hungarians thought this positioned them strongly when competing against Russia's largest EU neighbor for that business, since Poland's commitment to a single-payer system that included dental coverage had depressed quality among private clinics. (There is one potential advantage for Poland over other Eastern European countries: despite fewer opportunities to draw patients from neighboring countries by land—Berlin is at least a ninety-minute drive from the closest border crossing—it has more large cities served by international airports.)

Kútvölgyi Premium hired a Russian dentist who had studied in Hungary, and began subscribing to Russian-language fashion magazines. Despite its stated focus on French patients, Apollonia ensured that one of its nine dentists was a Russian who had previously worked in Moscow. Even the Four Seasons Hotel, located in the historic Gresham Palace building facing the Danube, invited a Russian operator to open a four-seat dental clinic on its property. Yet the timing was inauspicious for the clinic's owner: He was opening a business abroad just as his home country faced an economic crisis provoked by Russian incursions into Ukraine. The Russian owner closed up shop after six months, a consequence of a rapid decline of the ruble that effectively increased prices by nearly 20 percent. The Korchmároses, too, saw traffic from Russia to their Kútvölgyi Premium clinic fall by half in under three months, but the damage to their business was relatively contained.

Those economics led to a demand that was highly elastic. In early 2009, when the European Congress on Health Tourism held one of its regular conferences in Budapest, Bátorfi reported on the impact the global financial crisis had had on his business and those like it. The number of patients traveling from abroad had fallen by 30 percent, and those who did come were spending less: the average bill had fallen nearly in half, from 5,000 to 2,600 euros. Furthermore, the average age of patients was increasing, which Bátorfi concluded must mean that medical tourists were delaying treatments because of economic hardship.

Hungary, which despite its membership in the European Union had perpetually put off its adoption of the euro, saw its currency ravaged during the financial crisis. The forint lost over one-fifth of its value against the British pound over just a few months in late 2008. Dentists who as a service to customers simultaneously denominated their prices in multiple currencies found the fluctuations particularly unmanageable. After exchange rates stabilized, a freak natural disaster delayed any recovery. The 2010 eruption of Iceland's Eyjafjallajökull volcano, whose smoke disrupted European air travel for weeks, effectively put a halt to medical tourism from the British Isles and Scandinavia. Throughout this period, Hungarian banks tightened their credit, effectively asking for money back from dentists who had borrowed from them.

Without tax breaks or direct government subsidies, countries that committed to development through medical tourism exposed themselves to the same unpredictability as many conventional export-based economies. Hungarian dentists were able to recite the cautionary tale of neighboring Slovakia, where the dental sector similarly benefited from the introduction of low-cost flights to western Europe but saw its appeal diminished upon joining the euro in 2009. Prices quickly drifted closer to what one would expect to see in Vienna than in Sopron. "We are working with the same equipment, we have very highly qualified doctors, and the only difference is the cost of the human work—and that is because we're not in euros," says Miklós Rózsa, a senior EU project administrator working with Bátorfi's Medical Tourism Office to develop the Hungarian cluster. "As soon as we get euros, that gap will close."

As Greece wavered during the summer of 2015 about whether to depart the Eurozone, there were implications for ongoing efforts to promote "leisure travel to Greece with medical care, mainly for mild medical incidents," as the country's tourism minister, Olga Kefalogianni, had said in late 2013. She had just committed to a government strategy to make medical tourism a priority, focusing on rehabilitation and non-invasive treatment during which patients might prioritize pleasant surroundings. ("More than 1,000 tourists per year enjoy their dialysis holidays at MESOGEIOS Dialysis Centers in Greece," touts one Crete-based network of medical facilities.) The long-term disintegration of Greece's place in the European Union would likely end up setting back those plans, as western and northern Europeans could lose the ability to travel freely there. But if Greece departed the Eurozone, tourism would likely be among the first sectors to benefit as foreigners flocked to take advantage of a devalued drachma. "More medical and dental tourists to Greece could impact destinations such as Turkey, Hungary, and a host of former Russian states," wrote Ian Youngman in the *International Medical Travel Journal,* an online trade publication.

Even as Hungary's prime minister instruct Syrian refugees attempting to penetrate his borders as a pass-through to western and northern Europe to "please don't come," Viktor Orbán's policies continue to insouciantly promote Hungary as a destination for citizens of those other European countries seeking inexpensive dental care. Bátorfi and his advisers are hoping that the marketing machine they have developed with government funding—including the call center whose employees read the Fleet Street tabloids to enter the mind of an English would-be patient—can fend off efforts by regional rivals to encroach on a business he effectively built. "They can influence these people to pick Hungary, not to go to Poland, not to go to Bulgaria, not to go to Romania," says Szűcs.

Meanwhile, Bátorfi and Szűcs continue plotting a global strategy. "Maybe we will open several new big dental clinics backed with the Bátorfi model in the future," says Szűcs. "The know-how could be transferred to foreign places like Southeast Asia, like a knowledge transfer." It is not entirely clear that Szűcs—who says things like "the concept is not to sell Hungarian dentists themselves, but to sell Hungarian

dentistry"—has determined what exactly this would look
like, but he has already settled on a name for the brand: *By Béla Bátorfi.*

Epilogue

Even as Sofia residents began to take for granted the alabaster monument to foreign investment studding the capital's dismal low-rise skyline, Tokuda Hospital did not want to be mistaken for a local. A fifth anniversary celebration, in 2011, made a point of celebrating the hospital's unusual cross-cultural patrimony—the ceremony featured traditional Slavic music and the reception offered large platters of sushi next to European-style open-faced sandwiches. The anniversary party doubled as an opportunity for Tokuda to reveal that, after five years, it was time for some changes. Hospital administrators led guests on the inaugural tour of a new wing, filled with rooms more spacious and comfortable than anything Tokuda had been able to offer patients previously. The hospital administrators who stood poised with scissors at the new wing's ribbon-cutting were an even more diverse bunch than the hors d'oeuvres.

Alongside the Japanese and Bulgarian officials who had initially come together to make possible the Tokushukai Medical

Corporation's expansion into Europe were new colleagues from Britain. Tokuda had restructured its management board to welcome representatives of Addenbrooke's Hospital, a teaching institution affiliated with the University of Cambridge, in the United Kingdom. Addenbrooke's was one of many marquee hospitals around the world that had—through various types of partnerships, some of them little more than contracts to lease the brand to other hospital operators—expanded its reach overseas. The Cleveland Clinic has helped to develop facilities in Toronto, Vienna, and Abu Dhabi, and Harvard has seen its name on hospitals across five continents. (The university spun off the Harvard Medical International consulting business in 2008, to Partners HealthCare, in part because critics said its profit motive was incompatible with an educational mission.)

From its founding, Tokuda had taken pride in an institutional modesty that set it apart from hospitals operating with the spirit of tourism destinations more than that of medical providers. "PR and marketing with a lot of money was not a priority," says Iavor Drenski, Tokuda's executive director. "People are coming here because of our skillful doctors." In its first five years, Tokuda had drawn patients from beyond Eastern Europe and the Near East, with a few hundred patients yearly coming from Canada and the United States, without any concerted effort to market its services to them. (English was already often the lingua franca among Bulgarian personnel and Arabic-speaking patients.) Eventually Tokuda officials realized that, to improve their hospital's appeal to such patients, they needed not only to hire a publicist, but to think more seriously about packaging the patient experience.

108   In an effort to draw patients from farther afield, including
in North America, Tokuda has since opened an International
Ward, which offers hotel-like accommodations including living areas suited for family members of patients. The ward is
not as well-appointed as the Premier Royal Suite at Bangkok's
Bumrungrad (which scored first on TheRichest's list of "The 10
Most Luxurious Medical Tourism Destinations") or as osten-
tatiously opulent as anything from the Dubai-based company
promising that at its forthcoming "luxury hospital" in Mumbai
patients would travel by Rolls-Royce. The mere fact of an exclusive wing for foreigners—identified in some of the hospital's
materials, yet more grandiosely, as an "International Patient and
VIP Center"—only inflamed those who suspected that medical
tourism could itself be a luxury good.

    Yet the bulk of medical tourism today, at least beyond frivo-
lous cosmetic procedures, is not undertaken as an act of privi-
lege. Medical tourists are almost never people who have access
to the care they want at home at a price they can manage but
prefer to bring a sense of worldly adventure to the experience
of heart surgery. Rather, at their most vulnerable moments,
they are choosing to unmoor from familiar surroundings and
reposition themselves in a place where something as simple as
a nurse's instructions on what pills to take require an on-site
team of interpreters. Medical tourists are nearly always those
who have determined that the care they needed is, for some reason, unobtainable where they live.

    They are, nonetheless, frequently more advantaged than
citizens at their destination who lack the means to secure the
care they want at home. There is little evidence that medical

tourism causes that scarcity, however, or even exacerbates it. At its best, medical tourism is a form of wealth transfer that could help to subsidize the most costly aspects of maintaining a modern health-care system, particularly specialized infrastructure and doctors' wages. Even at its worst, medical tourism does not create new inequalities as much as magnify existing ones.

But foreigners who have sought to escape the dysfunctions of their home health-care systems remain a convenient scapegoat for local politicians unable to explain to their constituents the underlying causes of local scarcity—and what it would require to enact a policy that delivered a different result. If Bulgarians are upset that they linger on waiting lists for care at Tokuda or Nadezdha while foreigners are seen immediately, their blame would be better directed at the low percentage of federal spending used to finance the health-insurance system and the way it perpetuates a brain drain of Bulgarian specialists. Isn't the problem in Israel not that public hospitals pursue income from foreign patients but that they have the capacity to do so because their "official work day" ends at 3:00 p.m.?

Through the clarity of comparative advantage, medical tourism reveals that the shortcomings of one's local health-care options (at least in the developed world) are often not inevitable but the consequence of government policy. National health-care systems set priorities, by creating rules and incentives designed to produce low costs, guard skilled talent, and assure broad access or patient choice. Medical tourism is an act of personal defiance against the state's monopoly on decision-making about medical economics, and the trade-offs between access, quality, and cost that are at the heart of every national

110   system. Even systems that emphasize patient choice, like the
       American one, ensure selection among doctors or hospitals, not
       whether a patient would prefer a low price or short wait.

           For many, the only remaining choice is to travel—to be a
       flying body.

Acknowledgments

Jimmy So said he had several possible book topics that he hoped I would consider, but I didn't let him get beyond the first on his list before telling him I was in. As my editor at Columbia Global Reports, he has been a great collaborator from the outset of this project, as we schemed how and where to plot a story that would reveal the dynamics of such a variegated phenomenon in both interesting and surprising ways. I am much obliged to my agent Larry Weissman, and his partner Sascha Alper, for making the connection to Columbia Global Reports, and to Nicholas Lemann and Camille McDuffie there for effectively inventing a new journalistic format to encourage ambitious, worldly storytelling and bringing such high standards to it.

I was able to pull this project off only because my other professional guardians were so accommodating. My editor at Crown, Zack Wagman, was receptive when I asked for permission to work on a project for a potentially competitive publishing house; both he and Domenica Alioto were gracious as I pursued a far-flung distraction from the book I should have been working on for them. Similarly kind has been the team at Bloomberg Politics: John Heilemann, Mark Halperin, Josh Tyrangiel, Mike Nizza, Kelly Bare, Allison Hoffman, and especially John Homans. They gave me a pass to research corners of the cross-border trade in health care that they knew would yield no material in any way relevant to legislative debates over the Trans-Pacific Partnership or primary-season attacks on Obamacare. Over our seven-year relationship, the editors at *Monocle* have indulged many of my curiosities about quirky corners of globalization, including my inchoate interest in medical tourism: Tyler Brûlé, Andrew Tuck, and Steve Bloomfield. Lynn Vavreck first ventured that University of California, Los Angeles might be a good temporary home for me, and I am grateful to her for proposing a westward migration—and then to the Luskin School of Public Affairs' Bill Parent for making it happen and the Department of Political Science's Jeff Lewis for keeping me around. Further thanks to the staff of UCLA's Young Research Library for taking care of me ever since, and also the Hugh and Hazel Darling Law Library and Louise M. Darling Biomedical Library in particular.

On my Eastern European travels, two erstwhile interpreters—Eszter Kovács in Budapest and Sopron, and Teodora Kolarova in Sofia—both proved great company and were indispensable as I navigated clinics, hospital wards, and government ministries, all while ensuring I was well-fed on local delicacies. Back home, I owe a debt to Leigh Wilson for gamely brushing up her *magyar,* and patiently familiarizing herself with medical-financing jargon, to translate Hungarian media for me. Parisa

116   Roshan kindly read the manuscript and shared helpful editorial
advice. As ever, I am grateful to my kitchen cabinet—including James Burnett, Michael Schaffer, Jonathan Martin and April
White—for their friendship and counsel on this project and all
my other endeavors. Nothing would be possible without my
parents, Bella Brodzki and Henry Issenberg; my sister, Sarina
Issenberg; my aunt Gayle Brodzki; and my grandmother Olga
Issenberg, to whom this book is dedicated.

118   FURTHER READINGS

The most reader-friendly survey of medical tourism today is *Patients with Passports: Medical Tourism, Law, and Ethics* (Oxford University Press, 2014) by Harvard bioethicist I. Glenn Cohen, who writes with a particular eye to the legal and ethical challenges that the practice poses for individuals, governments, insurers, and medical providers.

Veteran foreign correspondent T. R. Reid's *The Healing of America: A Global Quest for Better, Cheaper, and Fairer Health Care* (Penguin, 2009) is a comparative health-economics textbook disguised as a self-help travelogue—and a vivid account of how sharply national health-care systems can differ, even across countries of similar economic means.

For a more thorough analysis of the tricky project of creating a one-size-fits-all policy for neighboring countries with seemingly irreconcilable systems, check out the 2010 report *Cross-Border Health Care in the European Union: Mapping and Analysing Practices and Policies*, published by the World Health Organization on behalf of the European Observatory on Health Systems and Policies, and edited by Matthias Wismar, Willy Palm, Josep Figueras, Kelly Ernst, and Ewout van Ginneken. (www.euro.who.int/__data/assets/pdf_file/00 04/135994/e94875.pdf)

Her March 2015 dispatch entitled "About Face" doesn't much explore South Korea's appeal to foreign patients, but the *New Yorker*'s Patricia Marx captures how much a global medical-tourism destination—in this case Seoul's emergence as "the world capital of plastic surgery"—is created by local factors, both current and historical. (www.newyorker.com/magazine/2015/03/23/about-face)

Tablet's Dimitri Linde describes how Israeli officials came to understand that an exodus of "transplant tourists" to overseas hospitals was a potential public-health crisis and set out to keep them donating their organs closer to home. The March 2014 article "Israel, a Leader in Transplant Tourism, Finds a Formula for Increasing Domestic Donations" shows a country acknowledging its control for creating an outbound supply and simultaneously pulling policy levers and pushing cultural buttons to limit it. (www.tabletmag.com/jewish-news-and-politics/164976/israel-organ-donation)

120   ENDNOTES

13   **First opened in 1980 with 200 beds:** "Who We Are," Bumrungrad International Hospital. https://www.bumrungrad.com/en/about-us/overview

13   **most notably, sexual reassignment surgery:** Prayuth Chokrungvaranont, Gennaro Selvaggi, Sirachai Jindarak, Apichai Angspatt, Pornthep Pungrasmi, Poonpismai Suwajo, and Preecha Tiewtranon, "The Development of Sex Reassignment Surgery in Thailand: A Social Perspective," *Scientific World Journal*, Volume 2014. http://dx.doi.org/10.1155/2014/182981

13   **patients representing 190 countries:** "How much experience does Bumrungrad have in treating international patients? What facilities does the hospital have in place specifically for international patients?" Bumrungrad International Hospital. https://www.bumrungrad.com/Hospital-FAQs/How-much-experience-does-Bumrungrad-have-in-treati

14   **branding Thailand the "Medical Hub of Asia":** Thailand: "Medical Hub of Asia," Thailand Board of Investment. http://thinkasiainvestthailand.com/download/medical.pdf

14   **Many X-rays taken in American clinics:** "Who's Reading Your X-Ray?" by Andrew Pollack, *New York Times*, Nov. 16, 2003. http://www.nytimes.com/2003/11/16/business/who-s-reading-your-x-ray.html

15   **Yemenis with heart disease often end up in India:** *Patients with Passports: Medical Tourism, Law and Ethics,* by I. Glenn Cohen (Oxford University Press, 2014).

20   **"Orbán is putting his people everywhere":** "Black sheep in the crimson dome," *Economist,* June 8, 2013. http://www.economist.com/news/europe/21579052-viktor-orban-once-again-accused-dismantling-rule-law-hungary-black-sheep

20   **"It is possible to get the money":** "Orbán fogorvosán át vezet az út az állami milliárdhoz," by Albert Ákos, *Origo*, Oct. 11, 2012. http://www.origo.hu/itthon/20121008-a-fogaszati turizmus-tamogatasara-szant-egy milliard-forint-tortenete.html

20   **"Bátorfi has been Orbán's dentist since 1992":** "Orbán fogászának szellemi leleménye az állami támogatás feltétele," by Júlia Gáti, *Heti Világgazdaság*, Jan. 28, 2012. http://hvg.hu/itthon/201204_tamogatas_a_fogturizmusnak_tomes_maskent

21   **"He is expanding into the entertainment business":** "Orbán fogorvosa most már sportszövetségi elnök is," *Heti Világgazdaság*, June 27, 2014.

http://hvg.hu/itthon/2014
0627_Orban_fogorvosa_most_mar_
sportszovetsegi

21 "What he lacked in bedside manner he made up for with efficiency": "Take a bite out of Budapest," by Johnny Morris, *Telegraph*, Nov. 18, 2006. http://www.telegraph.co.uk/travel/destinations/europe/hungary/737041/Take-a-bite-out-of-Budapest.html

23 "number of per-capita dentists in Hungary increased by 56 percent": "Why is Hungary the main destination country in dental tourism? Why do patients choose Hungary for dental care? Hungarian Case Study on dental care and patient flow," by Eszter Kovács, Gábor Szócska, Blanka Török, Károly Ragány, ECAB project (Grant agreement 242058), 2013. http://english.hsmtc.hu/site/wp-content/uploads/2013/02/Final_case_study_web.pdf

23 Hungary has more dentists per head of population than any other country: *The Complete Medical Tourist: Your Guide to Inexpensive and Safe Cosmetic and Medical Surgery Overseas*, by David Hancock (John Blake, 2006).

24 "A 2010 study by the country's central tax bureau": "Hungary aims at bigger bite of dental tourism," by Krisztián Kummer, *Budapest Business Journal*, July 9, 2012. http://bbj.hu/business/hungary-aims-at-bigger-bite-of-dental-tourism_63662

25 "In 2011, he was informed": 121
"Eltiltották hivatásától Angliában Orbán Viktor fogorvosát," *Origo*, May 19, 2011. http://www.origo.hu/itthon/20110519-eltiltottak-hivatasa-gyakorlasatol-angliaban-batorfi-belat-a-magyar-fogturizmust-nepszerusito.html

25 the suspension was rescinded: "Már nincs brit tiltólistán Orbán fogorvosa," *Válasz*, May 21, 2011. http://valasz.hu/itthon/a-turistak-altalaban-elegedettek-38005

28 "It has often been said": *Value for Money in the Health Services* by Brian Abel-Smith (Heinemann, 1976).

28 Bismarck had begun experimenting: *The Healing of America: A Global Quest for Better, Cheaper, and Fairer Health Care* by T.R. Reid (Penguin Press, 2009).

29 "Governments have a responsibility for the health": *Declaration of Alma Ata,* World Health Organization. http://www.euro.who.int/__data/assets/pdf_file/0009/113877/E93944.pdf

30 Today approximately sixty countries: "The political economy of universal health coverage" by David Stuckler, Andrea B Feigl, Sanjay Basu, Martin McKee, Background Paper for the Global Symposium on Health Systems Research, 2010. http://healthsystemsresearch.org/hsr2010/images/stories/8political_economy.pdf

122   31   **shared patterns of industrial-ization:** "What Is Policy Convergence and What Causes It?" by Colin J. Bennett. *British Journal of Political Science* Vol. 21, No. 2 (1991). http://healthsystemsresearch.org/hsr2010/images/stories/8political_economy.pdf

31   **a model they call convergence theory:** "Globalization and Policy Convergence," by Daniel W. Drezner, *International Studies Review* Vol. 3, No. 1 (Spring, 2001). http://daniel drezner.com/research/policy convergence.pdf

31   **"towards the Bev-marck or Bis-eridge model":** "Bismarck vs. Beveridge: is there increasing convergence between health financing systems?" presentation by Joseph Kutzin at the 1st annual meeting of SBO network on health expenditure, November 2011. http://www.oecd.org/gov/budgeting/49095378.pdf

34   **specifically singled out:** North American Free Trade Agreement, Part 5, Chapter 11, Section A, Article 1101, Clause 4. http://www.sice.oas.org/trade/nafta/chap-111.asp

35   **The Emirates' first:** "Hope for patients as kidney transplant centre opens in Dubai," by Jennifer Bell, *National,* Jan. 19, 2014. http://www.thenational.ae/uae/health/hope-for-patients-as-kidney-transplant-centre-opens-in-dubai

37   **considered it as a separate profession:** *Social Medicine in Eastern Europe: The Organization of Health Services and the Education of Medical Personnel in Czechoslovakia, Hungary, and Poland* by E. Richard Weinerman (Harvard University Press, 1969).

39   **site of the Pan-European Picnic:** "The picnic that changed European history" by Christian Erdei, *Deutsche Welle,* Aug. 19, 2014. http://dw.com/p/JDcu

42   **1,371 private dental facilities:** "Why is Hungary the main destination country in dental tourism? Why do patients choose Hungary for dental care? Hungarian Case Study on dental care and patient flow," by Eszter Kovács, Gábor Szócska, Blanka Török, Károly Ragány, ECAB project (Grant agreement 242058), 2013. http://english.hsmtc.hu/site/wp-content/uploads/2013/02/Final_case_study_web.pdf

42   **number of foreign students:** "Why is Hungary the main destination country in dental tourism? Why do patients choose Hungary for dental care? Hungarian Case Study on dental care and patient flow," by Eszter Kovács, Gábor Szócska, Blanka Török, Károly Ragány, ECAB project (Grant agreement 242058), 2013. http://english.hsmtc.hu/site/wp-content/uploads/2013/02/Final_case_study_web.pdf

44   **around 80 percent of dentists:** "Why is Hungary the main destination country in dental tourism? Why do patients choose Hungary

for dental care? Hungarian Case Study on dental care and patient flow," by Eszter Kovács, Gábor Szócska, Blanka Török, Károly Ragány, ECAB project (Grant agreement 242058), 2013. http://english.hsmtc.hu/site/wp-content/uploads/2013/02/Final_case_study_web.pdf

44 Since 600 A.D.: "A Brief Historical Perspective on Dental Implants, Their Surface Coatings and Treatments," by Celeste M. Abraham, *Open Dentistry Journal*, May 2014. http://www.ncbi.nlm.nih.gov/pmc/articles/PMC4040928/pdf/TODENTJ-8-50.pdf

48 "Dental tourism will play": "Orbán fogászát eltiltották Angliában," by E.S.P., *Blikk,* May 19, 2011. http://www.blikk.hu/blikk_aktualis/orban-fogaszat-eltiltottak-angliaban-2052667

50 Most subsidies per capita: *EU Funds in Central and Eastern Europe, Progress Report 2007-2013,* by KPMG Central and Eastern Europe, 2014. http://www.kpmg.com/SI/en/Issues AndInsights/ArticlesPublications/Documents/EU-Funds-in-Central-and-Eastern-Europe.pdf

50 Some have likened to the Marshall Plan: "Cohesion Policy and other EU assistance programmes in 2014-2020," by Jan Jedlička Česká and Katarzyna Rzentarzewska (Erste Corporate Banking, May 2014). https://www.erstegroup.com/en/Downloads/b4bc0801-aeb3-423e-80ec-1ed1

00e1164a/pi20140311-Report.pdf;GP JSESSIONID=34j0Vz3FnL2xkHTV5v SqzxSvqPLGn9Gvb2KGyQyvQ7slljfZ TQ9N!-1494673580

53 below the European Union average: "Why is Hungary the main destination country in dental tourism? Why do patients choose Hungary for dental care? Hungarian Case Study on dental care and patient flow," by Eszter Kovács, Gábor Szócska, Blanka Török, Károly Ragány, ECAB project (Grant agreement 242058), 2013. http://english.hsmtc.hu/site/wp-content/uploads/2013/02/Final_case_study_web.pdf

59 St. John's had only five departments: "Szent János Kórház és Észak-budai Egyesített Kórházak: Történet." http://www.janoskorhaz.hu/tortenet/

59 number of per-capita hospital beds: *Social Medicine in Eastern Europe: The Organization of Health Services and the Education of Medical Personnel in Czechoslovakia,Hungary, and Poland,* by E. Richard Weinerman (Harvard University Press, 1969).

60 Nearly all medicine in Hungary: *The Planning of Health Services: Studies in Eight European Countries,* edited by G. McLachlan (World Health Organization, 1980)

61 By 1980, Hungary had: *Implementing Health Financing Reform: Lessons from countries in transition,*

124   edited by Joseph Kutzin, Cheryl Cashin, Melitta Jakab (European Observatory on Health Systems and Policies, 2010). http://www.euro.who.int/__data/assets/pdf_file/0014/120164/E94240.pdf

61   doctors were subsidized through a practice: *Health law and Health Administration in Hungary,* by Adam Rixer (Patrocinium Kiadó, 2014). http://real.mtak.hu/16307/1/Health%20Law%20and%20Health%20Administration%20in%20Hungary%5B1%5D.pdf

61   4,000 out of Hungary's 25,000 doctors: *Implementing Health Financing Reform: Lessons from countries in transition,* edited by Joeseph Kutzin, Cheryl Cashin, Melitta Jakab (European Observatory on Health Systems and Policies, 2010). http://www.euro.who.int/__data/assets/pdf_file/0014/120164/E94240.pdf

68   In 2010, a reporter: "Haaretz probe: Israel gives medical tourists perks denied to citizens," by Dan Even and Maya Zinshtein, *Haaretz,* Nov. 18, 2010. http://www.haaretz.com/print-edition/news/haaretz-probe-israel-gives-medical-tourists-perks-denied-to-citizens-1.325275

68   Bloomberg in 2014 ranked: "Most Efficient Health Care 2014: Countries," Bloomberg Visual Data. http://www.bloomberg.com/visual-data/best-and-worst/most-efficient-health-care-2014-countries

70   Al-Jazeera noted that Nigerians: "Nigeria's weak health sector confronts Ebola," by Maram Mazen, Al-Jazeera, Sept. 18 2014. http://www.aljazeera.com/news/africa/2014/09/nigeria-weak-health-sector-confronts-ebola-2014915917268515.html

71   more than 90 percent of Nigerians: "Nigeria Operating 19th Century Health System," Mustapha Danesi interviewed by Jide Akintunde, Nigeria Development & Finance Forum. http://www.nigeriadevelopmentandfinanceforum.org/PolicyDialogue/Dialogue.aspx?Edition=49

72   An undercover team from Channel 2: "Medical tourists in Israel given needless surgery - for money, doctors accuse" by Ido Efrati, *Haaretz,* Feb. 18, 2015. http://www.haaretz.com/business/.premium-1.642937

73   "will be seriously harmed": "New rules could kill medical tourism, hospitals charge" by Ronny Linder-Ganz, *Haaretz,* Dec. 29, 2013. http://www.haaretz.com/business/.premium-1.565932

75   In 1996, Manfred Molenaar: *Manfred Molenaar and Barbara Fath-Molenaar v Allgemeine Ortskrankenkasse Baden-Württemberg,* Case C-160/96, European Court Reports 1998 I-00843. http://curia.europa.eu/juris/showPdf.jsf;jsessionid=9ea7d0f130de711e27b3fc8940a99000c65421b8cd9d.e34KaxiLc3eQc40LaxqMbN4OaNuLe0?docid=43655&pageIndex=0&doc

lang=EN&dir=&occ=first&part=1&
cid=116293

75 **The following year:** *Friedrich
Jauch v Pensionsversicherungsanstalt
der Arbeiter,* Case C-215/99, European
Court Reports 2001 I-01901. http://
eur-lex.europa.eu/legal-content/EN
/TXT/?uri=CELEX:61999CJ0215

76 **In 2001, the court further ruled:**
*Ghislain Leclere and Alina Deaconescu
v Caisse nationale des prestations
familiales,* Case C-43/99, European
Court Reports 2001 I-04265.
http://eur-lex.europa.eu/legal-
content/EN/TXT/?uri=CELEX:61999
CJ0043

77 **"Union action shall respect":**
Consolidated version of the Treaty
on the Functioning of the European
Union - Protocols - Annexes
-Declarations annexed to the Final
Act of the Intergovernmental
Conference, which adopted the Treaty
of Lisbon, signed on Dec. 13, 2007.
http://eur-lex.europa.eu/legal-content/
EN/TXT/?uri=celex:12012E/TXT

77 **"The** *Molenaar* **and** *Jauch* **cases
thus":** "Welfare States and Social
Europe," by Dorte Singdbjerg
Martinsen, in *Social Services of General
Interest in the EU,* edited by Ulla
Neergaard, Erika Szyszczak, Johan
Willem van de Gronden, Markus
Krajewski (T.M.C. Asser Press, 2013).

78 **"resolution to begin the
process":** "Coordination of social
security systems ***II," P5_TA(2004)

0293, European Parliament. http://
www.europarl.europa.eu/sides
/getDoc.do?pubRef=-//EP//
NONSGML+TA+P5-TA-2004-
0293+0+DOC+PDF+V0//
EN

78 **"medically necessary, state-
provided":** "European Health
Insurance Card," European
Commission. http://ec.europa.eu/
social/main.jsp?catId=559

80 **Only 1 percent of Europe's:**
"Q&A: Patients' Rights in Cross-
Border Healthcare," European
Commission. http://europa.eu/
rapidpress-release_MEMO-13-
918_en.htm

88 **Hezbollah targeted an Israeli
tour bus:** "Bulgaria Implicates
Hezbollah in July Attack on Israelis,"
by Nicholas Kulish, Eric Schmitt,
and Matthew Brunwasser,
New York Times, Feb. 5, 2013. http://
www.nytimes.com/2013/02/06/
world/europe/bulgaria-implicates-
hezbollah-in-deadly-israeli-bus-
blast.html

89 **Swedes receive an average of
about three thousand euros
monthly:** "Pensions at a Glance 2013,"
Organisation for Economic
Co-operation and Development, Nov.
26, 2013. http://www.oecd-ilibrary.
org/finance-and-investment/pensions-
at-a-glance-2013_pension_glance-
2013-en

126

96 Italy and Turkey: "IFFS Surveillance 2013," International Federation of Fertility Societies, Oct. 2013. https://c.ymcdn.com/sites/iffs.site-ym.com/resource/resmgr/iffs_surveillance_09-19-13.pdf

97 In November 2014: "Turkey reveals new economic plan to boost economy," by Feyza Süsal and Bahattin Gönültaş, Anadolu Agency, Nov. 6, 2014. http://www.aa.com.tr/en/economy/416106--turkey-reveals-new-economic-plan-to-boost-economy

102 when the European Congress on Health Tourism held: "The Challenge Facing the Medical Tourism Industry," *International Medical Travel Journal*, Apr. 14, 2009. http://www.imtj.com/articles/2009/blog-challenge-facing-medical-tourism-industry-40145/

103 "leisure travel to Greece": "Kefalogianni: Development Of Medical Tourism In Greece Is A Priority," *Greek Travel Pages,* Dec. 12, 2013. http://news.gtp.gr/2013/12/12/kefalogianni-development-medical-tourism-greece-priority/

104 "More medical and dental tourists to Greece": "Greece Crisis. . . The Implications for Greek Medical Tourism," by Ian Youngman, *International Medical Tourism Journal,* July 2015. http://www.imtj.com/articles/2015/greece-crisis-greek-medical-tourism-implications-40206/

107 the university spun off: "Goodbye to HMI," *Harvard Magazine,* May-June 2008. http://harvardmagazine.com/2008/05/good-bye-to-hmi.html

108 which scored first: "The 10 Most Luxurious Medical Tourism Destinations," by Octavia Drughi, The Richest, April 22, 2014. http://www.therichest.com/luxury/the-10-most-luxurious-medical-tourism-destinations/

108 Dubai-based company promising: "Rolls Royces, movies: private India hospitals go luxe for growth," by Zeba Siddiqui and Aditya Kalra, Reuters, May 28, 2015. http://www.reuters.com/article/2015/05/28/us-india-health-luxury-idUSKBN0OC2QA20150528

Columbia Global Reports is a publishing imprint from Columbia University that commissions authors to do original on-site reporting around the globe on a wide range of issues. The resulting novella-length books offer new ways to look at and understand the world that can be read in a few hours. Most readers are curious and busy. Our books are for them.

globalreports.columbia.edu